Post COVID-19 Complications and Management

Anant Mohan • Saurabh Mittal
Editors

Post COVID-19 Complications and Management

Springer

Editors
Anant Mohan
Department of Pulmonary, Critical Care and Sleep Medicine
All India Institute of Medical Sciences
New Delhi, India

Saurabh Mittal
Department of Pulmonary, Critical Care and Sleep Medicine
All India Institute of Medical Sciences
New Delhi, India

ISBN 978-981-19-4409-3 ISBN 978-981-19-4407-9 (eBook)
https://doi.org/10.1007/978-981-19-4407-9

This Springer imprint is published by the registered company Springer Nature Singapore Pte Ltd.
The registered company address is: 152 Beach Road, #21-01/04 Gateway East, Singapore 189721, Singapore

Foreword

The COVID-19 pandemic has severely affected the healthcare system across the globe and caused significant morbidity and mortality. The occurrence and importance of post-COVID-19 sequelae was realized later in the pandemic when it was noted that a sizable proportion of patients continued to suffer from various symptoms even weeks to months after recovering from the acute episode. Further, these complications were observed in multiple organ systems and not just the respiratory tract. The current understanding of these complications is limited by the sparse literature regarding the recognition, diagnosis, and treatment of various sequelae. Moreover, multidisciplinary efforts are required to manage these patients as the complications are variable in terms of location as well as severity.

In the above context, this book is a timely and important endeavor that deals with all aspects of post-COVID complications, with emphasis on all relevant body systems, and their appropriate management. This book will help clinicians understand the recognition of various post-covid sequelae and their management. This will also be a useful reference source for academicians, researchers, and students to identify research gaps that need further exploration.

I congratulate all the authors and editors for their dedication and hard work in bringing out this comprehensive book on a contemporary and important topic.

Delhi, India

Vinod Paul

Foreword

The COVID-19 pandemic has affected millions of individuals around the globe and has overwhelmed the healthcare systems. Although lungs are the most commonly affected by the SARS-CoV-2 virus, it is now known that this disease affects almost all body systems, thus making its management even more challenging. Significant morbidity and mortality have been caused not just by the acute manifestations, but also by the long-term complications, what is now called as post-covid or long-covid. While the acute manifestations have been studied better, we are still struggling to recognize and treat the various post-covid manifestations seen after the initial infection. The research in this area is as yet limited, and most of the work has focused on one or few organ systems only rather than on multisystem manifestations. A holistic knowledge of various post-covid complications or sequelae is therefore essential for general physicians, internists, and specialists alike. In this regard, this book is likely to serve as a useful and timely reference tool as it summarizes the currently available evidence for post-COVID manifestations and provides a practical approach to dealing with them. All the authors have tried to synthesize the text, which is easy to read and can be applied to individual patient care. I appreciate the efforts of all the authors and editors for their hard work and wish them success in further such endeavors in the future.

Delhi, India

Randeep Guleria

Foreword

It gives me immense pleasure to write the foreword for this book on post-COVID complications. The COVID-19 pandemic started in late 2019 and continues to wreak havoc globally, having caused huge loss of life and putting immense pressure on health services. Although majority of infections recovered without sequelae, a large number of patients reported delayed complications over the subsequent weeks to months. Initially thought to affect only the respiratory system, gradually it became evident that post-covid complications may affect several organ systems. Unfortunately, the mechanism and clinical course of these complications is still not properly understood, thereby hampering appropriate management.

With this background, a comprehensive coverage of various post-covid complications was definitely considered necessary, and this book provides detailed information on these complications in multiple body systems and outlines a management plan for them. This is surely going to be a reliable and scientific reference for all healthcare professionals who deal with covid-related complications. I congratulate all the authors and editors for their hard work and convey my best wishes for many more future endeavors.

Delhi, India

Balram Bhargava

Preface

Even after 2 years, the COVID-19 pandemic continues globally with a waxing-waning course, already having caused considerable suffering and disease. Although initially thought of as an ailment limited to the respiratory tract, it is clear that the disease has a multisystem dimension. The extra-pulmonary manifestations have often resulted in unpredictable and unexpected adverse outcomes, such as cardiovascular and thrombotic complications. As the experience with COVID-19 grows and we have longer follow-ups of patients after initial infection, numerous long-term sequelae have also been recognized affecting various organ systems to a variable degree. While most of these sequelae are fortunately not life-threatening, others, such as irreversible pulmonary fibrosis have caused significant morbidity and mortality.

It is now evident that post-COVID sequelae are likely to be an important new entity for medical professionals of all specialties. It is, therefore, essential that we keep ourselves informed regarding the numerous long-term manifestations of COVID-19. With this thought in mind, this book has been written to cover the various complications affecting different organ systems following COVID-19. Our attempt has been to cover all relevant systems and provides a comprehensive clinical reference. The book is intended not only for internists but also for various specialties and sub-specialties who are likely to encounter COVID-19-related sequelae in their area of expertise. In addition, this will be a valuable sourcebook for post-graduates in various specialties. An attempt has been made to keep the text crisp but up to date with the currently available knowledge. Adequate referencing has been provided although the book is not meant to be an exhaustive source of references.

We gratefully acknowledge the support from the Springer (India) team and all the eminent faculty who contributed chapters of their specialty. We hope this book will benefit the readers and be enjoyed by them as much as we enjoyed bringing it out.

New Delhi, India — Anant Mohan
New Delhi, India — Saurabh Mittal

Contents

COVID-19: An Overview

1

Harish Moorjani and S. K. Gupta

The coronavirus disease 2019 (COVID-19) is a viral infection caused by a novel severe acute respiratory syndrome coronavirus 2 (SARS-CoV-2), which has emerged as a global pandemic leading to a massive loss of human life worldwide due to its high transmissibility.

1.1 Epidemiology

Epidemiology assumes a vital role during a pandemic. A quick analysis of data regarding infection, hospitalizations, recoveries, and deaths helps frame policy and guidelines. Model-based projections are useful guiding tools in the initial days or weeks of a pandemic; however, real-world data assumes greater significance as the pandemic evolves.

1.2 The Virus and Its Variants

At the beginning of the pandemic, a novel coronavirus was identified as the causative organism for a few cases of a particular type of pneumonia noticed in Wuhan, China, in 2019. The disease soon spread in China, and later the contagion engulfed the whole world to be declared a pandemic by WHO on March 11, 2020. In February 2020, the World Health Organization labeled the disease COVID-19, and the virus causing the disease was named SARS-CoV-2 by the experts. The enveloped

H. Moorjani (✉)
Clinical Assistant Professor of Medicine, New York Medical College, Valhalla, NY, USA

S. K. Gupta
GS Medical College, Pilkhuwa, UP, India

Max Super Speciality Hospital, Delhi, India

A. Mohan, S. Mittal (eds.), *Post COVID-19 Complications and Management*,
https://doi.org/10.1007/978-981-19-4407-9_1

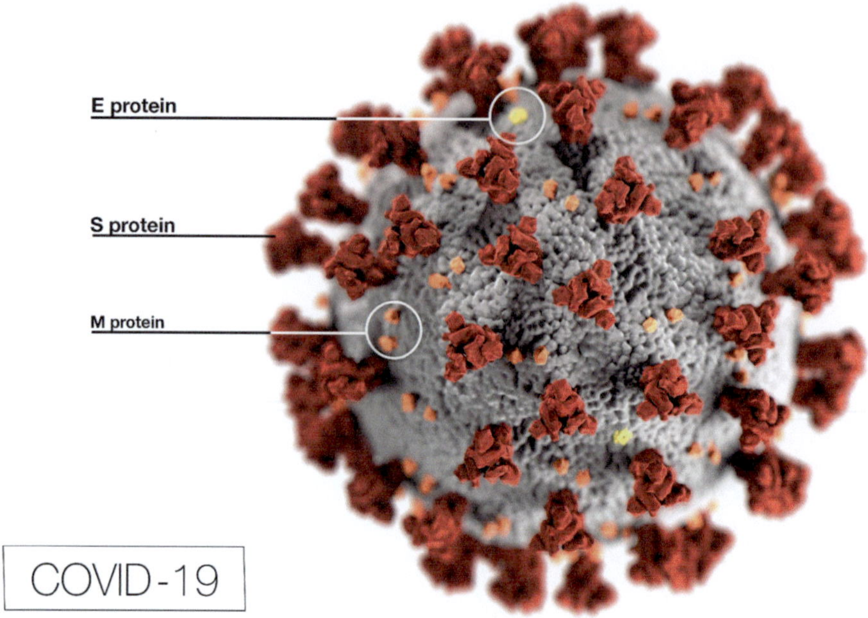

Fig. 1.1 Protein structure of SARS-CoV-2 (Image courtesy: Centers for Disease Control and Prevention)

positive-stranded RNA virus enters the host cell through ACE-2 receptors by latching its spike proteins (Fig. 1.1).

SARS-CoV-2, like other RNA viruses including influenza, is prone to making errors in its genetic code during replication, resulting in mutations. New mutations can produce variants which have properties different from the original strain. When any variant becomes more virulent, showing faster transmission or causing severe disease overriding the existing immunity, it is called a variant of concern. The SARS-CoV-2, within 2 months of its origin, mutated to a variant carrying the D614G spike protein mutation, and the mutant was called G614. The G614 variant had a fitness advantage and soon became the globally dominant form of SARS-CoV-2. In the absence of any effective antiviral drug, the virus evolves to more virulent forms. Notable changes in the virus have been named Alpha, Beta, Gamma, and Delta variants by WHO in May 2021. Variants should not be confused with Alpha, Beta, Gamma, and Delta families of coronavirus. All variants of SARS-CoV-2 belong to the Beta coronavirus family. The Alpha variant was detected in England (Kent) as early as September 2020. It was 43–90% more transmissible than pre-existing variants of SARS-CoV-2 [1]. The virus further mutated with significant double mutation evolving into Delta variant. The P681R mutation in the Delta variant speeds up the spread of SARS-CoV-2 from cell to cell. It was first detected in India in October 2020 and rapidly spread across the globe within the next few months. Beta is the South African variant, and Gamma is the Brazilian variant. On

November 24, 2021, a new variant of SARS-CoV-2, B.1.1.529, was reported to the WHO. This new variant was first detected in specimens collected on November 11, 2021, in Botswana and on November 14, 2021, in South Africa. On November 26, 2021, the WHO named the B.1.1.529 Omicron.

As per WHO, more than 438 million cases and 5.96 million deaths have been reported worldwide; however, the true incidence based on serosurveys is up to ten times higher as a large number of cases remain underreported due to subclinical infections, poor testing, and lack of reporting [2].

1.3 Infection

Having established a reservoir in humans, the disease spreads from person to person. Respiratory droplets, expelled by the infected person on coughing, talking, or sneezing and inhaled by subjects within close range of 2 m, remain the primary source of spread. Direct contact of infected hands with mucus membranes in eyes, nose, and mouth can also lead to infection. However, surface contact through fomites is no longer considered an important source of transmission. On the other hand, airborne transmission is now considered an important mode of transmission. Although viral particles can be detected in body specimens such as semen, stool, tears, and blood, transmission via these non-respiratory means remains uncertain [3].

The incubation period, defined as the time of exposure until the onset of symptoms, averages 4 to 5 days but could range between 2 and 14 days.

Individuals remain most infectious between 2 days before and 1 day after the onset of symptoms; contagiousness declines within 7 days of onset of symptoms irrespective of virus levels in the nose. Close contact for long durations increases the risk of transmission, especially in immunity naïve subjects. It can take a couple of days after exposure to COVID-19 to become infected with the virus and for the polymerase chain reaction (PCR) test to become positive. Hence, if the test is negative 24 h after exposure, the Centers for Disease Control and Prevention (CDC) recommends a retesting 5 to 7 days later even if the individual is asymptomatic. However, testing strategies continue to get updated depending on the disease burden.

1.4 Prevention

Preventive measures include: maintaining a physical distance of more than 2 m, wearing an appropriate mask, frequent hand-washing, and using alcohol-based sanitizers with at least 60% or 70% alcohol. Mass vaccination remains the key to pandemic control and disease eradication. Postexposure precautions include monitoring for symptoms in quarantine for 10–14 days, especially for unvaccinated individuals. Fully vaccinated/immunized individuals should be exempted from quarantine but advised to get tested 3–5 days after exposure and wear a mask in public until the test is negative, or for 14 days [4].

1.5 Clinical Features

The clinical spectrum of SARS-CoV-2 infection ranges from asymptomatic infection to critical and fatal illness. Patients should be suspected of having COVID-19 when they present with compatible symptoms, or have had recent close contact with a confirmed patient with COVID-19. The proportion of infections that remain asymptomatic is unclear. In longitudinal studies, the follow-up to identify patients testing positive who develop symptoms is sometimes not performed. Nevertheless, seroprevalence studies suggest that up to 40% of infections are asymptomatic [5]. Most symptomatic infections are mild. However, severe disease (hypoxia and pneumonia) has been reported in 15 to 20% of symptomatic infections; these can occur in patients of any age but usually occurs in adults with advanced age or in persons with underlying medical comorbidities like diabetes, hypertension, chronic obstructive pulmonary disease (COPD), obesity, cardiac diseases, chronic kidney disease (CKD), etc. In addition, some patients with initially mild symptoms may progress to severe illness over the course of days.

Fever, cough, myalgia, and headache remain the most common symptoms. Diarrhea, sore throat, and loss of smell and taste may be other common presenting complaints [6, 7]. Seasonal viral infections, including flu and common cold, may have a similar presentation. However, there are no pathognomic features that distinguish COVID-19 from other respiratory infections.

Asymptomatic individuals, who get tested following close contact with a patient of COVID-19 or for some other reason, should be advised careful monitoring and isolation. Patients with any signs and symptoms of COVID-19 (e.g., cough, fever, sore throat, malaise, headache, body ache, diarrhea, loss of taste and smell) but who maintain oxygen saturation > 94% on room air and do not have any evidence of pneumonitis on chest imaging are classified as mild disease. These patients can be monitored at home. On the other hand, individuals with mild disease but with comorbidities such as diabetes, hypertension, coronary artery disease, chronic kidney disease, or COPD and who are solid organ transplant recipients, are more than 65 years, or are on immunosuppressive therapy may require close in-hospital monitoring due to higher risk of progression to severe disease.

Patients showing any symptom of disease along with bilateral ground-glass opacities/consolidation on X-ray chest or lung ultrasound, or hypoxia manifested by SpO2 less than or equal to 94%, are labeled as having moderate disease and need hospitalization. Individuals with SpO2 < 90%, requiring mechanical ventilation with PaO2/FiO2 of 151–300 mm Hg, or respiratory rate > 30 breaths/min are classified as having severe disease and require ICU care.

1.6 Happy Hypoxia in COVID-19

Blood oxygen saturation (SpO2) for a healthy person remains in the range of 97 to 100% irrespective of age. Decline in SpO2 below 94% (or even earlier) leads to symptoms such as fatigue, air hunger, respiratory discomfort, and breathlessness.

Surprisingly, however, some patients with COVID-19 pneumonia do not demonstrate these manifestations even at very low SpO2 and may appear very comfortable. This situation is termed as happy hypoxia. The SARS-CoV-2, on one hand, causes hypoxic damage, while on the other, it blunts the body's defense mechanism to detect and repair the damage. Persistent hypoxia in COVID-19 may impair tissue oxygenation and lead to multi-organ failure. Pulse oximetry is the only noninvasive way to detect hypoxia both in home and hospital settings. Therefore, no patient should be treated at home without a suitable pulse oximeter, even in remote areas.

Apart from the above clinical symptoms and signs, some laboratory parameters such as lymphopenia, deranged NLR (neutrophil/lymphocyte ratio), elevated D-dimer, and elevated inflammatory markers as C-reactive protein (CRP) and LDH have been associated with severe COVID-19 and worse outcomes [8].

1.7 Complications

In patients with severe disease, development of hypoxemic respiratory failure leading to acute respiratory distress syndrome (ARDS) is the major complication. Other complications include pulmonary thromboembolism, myocarditis, acute renal failure, and inflammatory complications. In addition, the multisystem inflammatory syndrome can occur in children. About 40% of patients may have persistent symptoms following acute COVID-19 called "long COVID," which remains the primary focus of the subsequent chapters in this book.

1.8 Diagnosis of COVID-19

The possibility of COVID-19 should be considered in all patients with acute respiratory symptoms with or without fever, especially in cases where no other etiology can be identified. All symptomatic patients with suspected COVID-19 should undergo testing for SARS-CoV-2.

1.8.1 Nucleic Acid Amplification Test (NAAT)

Nucleic acid amplification test (NAAT) with a reverse transcription-polymerase chain reaction (RT PCR) assay is the preferred diagnostic test to detect SARS-CoV-2 RNA from the upper respiratory tract in patients with suspected COVID-19.

NAATs detect SARS-CoV-2 RNA in patient specimens and are highly specific. Although these tests can detect very low levels of viral RNA, their sensitivity depends on the type and quality of the specimen obtained, the duration of illness at the time of testing, and the specific assay. However, a positive NAAT for SARS-CoV-2 is confirmatory for the diagnosis of COVID-19. Conversely, false-negative results may occur in 2 to 40% of patients. Therefore, in symptomatic individuals with high suspicion for COVID-19, an initial negative NAAT result should be confirmed with a repeat test. In hospitalized patients with lower respiratory tract disease, performing NAAT on lower respiratory tract specimens like BAL (bronchoalveolar lavage) may yield better results.

Testing asymptomatic persons should include close contacts of a COVID-19 case, screening in long-term care facilities, shelters for the homeless, and in hospitalized patients in high-prevalence regions. Postexposure testing should be done 5 days after exposure, although the optimal timing is not established.

1.8.2 Rapid Antigen Test

Tests that detect SARS-CoV-2 antigen can be performed rapidly and at the point of care. Rapid antigen tests (RAT) have around 56% sensitivity compared to 72% sensitivity of RT-PCR-based tests [9].

However, antigen testing may be the initial test used in resource-poor settings. They can be helpful in the rapid diagnosis of patients soon after the onset of symptoms. Antigen tests also find a place in serial screening for infection in congregate settings. Rapid antigen test detects S gene, and since many mutants have a deletion of S gene, these are not picked up by the rapid antigen test. On the other hand, RT-PCR detects the ORF and N gene in addition to the S gene. Since antigen tests have lower sensitivity than RT-PCR, a negative RAT should usually be confirmed with RT-PCR.

1.8.3 Serologic Tests

Serologic tests are used to detect antibodies to SARS-CoV-2 in the blood in order to help identify patients who previously had exposure to this virus. However, detectable antibodies generally take at least 2 weeks to develop; thus, serologic tests have little utility for diagnosis in the acute care setting. In addition, serologic assays have variable performance among various company kits. They also have poor positive predictive value in low seroprevalence settings. In addition, serologic assay values may not always correlate with immunity. Sometimes, serologic testing like anti-S antibodies or anti-nucleocapsid antigen antibodies may be the only option left for the diagnosis, especially in patients presenting with symptoms for at least 2 weeks. However, serologic tests may not differentiate acute infection from past infection. Results of serologic testing may also be affected by prior vaccination, while previous COVID-19 vaccination does not influence NAAT or antigen test results. Most serologic tests target the nucleocapsid protein; only serologic tests for spike protein can detect antibody response to currently available mRNA and vector-based vaccines, but they cannot distinguish a vaccine response from a prior infection.

1.9 Management of COVID-19

The spectrum of COVID-19 disease ranges from asymptomatic infection to mild flu-like symptoms to severe pneumonia with ARDS and multi-organ failure. So, our understanding of COVID-19 disease as well as optimizing its management continues to evolve.

The management of adult patients with acute COVID-19 in the outpatient setting (<12 weeks after onset of illness) includes early and appropriate risk stratification, self-care advice, telehealth and clinic management, timely referral to the emergency department (ED), and posthospital discharge care. The approach is guided by increasing clinical experience in the rapidly evolving scenario of evidence-based medicine. Therefore, clinicians should consider the individual patient's clinical and social circumstances to formulate a personal COVID-19 care plan.

The initial clinical evaluation includes assessment of risk factors for progressive disease (see below), oxygenation status, severity of dyspnea, and the patient's general medical condition to determine whether intensive care is required or outpatient care is sufficient.

The patients with the following symptoms/signs should be referred to the ED for further management:

- Shortness of breath (at rest, and inability to speak complete sentences)
- Saturation on room air of ≤90%, regardless of the severity of dyspnea
- Mental status (confusion, change in behavior, drowsiness) or signs and symptoms of inadequate perfusion (hypotension, cyanosis, cardiac chest pain)

Patients can be managed at home without in-person evaluation if they are able to maintain daily clinical contact, promptly report worsening symptoms, and self-isolate for the duration of illness. Telemedicine follow-up depends upon their risk for severe disease and the severity of symptoms.

During home isolation, patients should be provided clear instructions for self-care. The use of paracetamol for fever control, antitussive remedies for relief of cough, and adequate bed rest should be emphasized. For patients with early, symptomatic COVID-19 and risk factors for progression to severe illness (Table 1.1), treatment with monoclonal antibody infusion has been suggested, preferably within 7 to 10 days of symptom onset. Options available through emergency use authorization include casirivimab-imdevimab, sotrovimab, and bamlanivimab-etesevimab and may reduce the risk of progression to severe disease [10].

Several other therapies are being studied for the treatment of COVID-19, but none have been proven in asymptomatic or mild disease and should be prescribed only in a clinical trial setting. In nonhospitalized patients, the routine use of systemic corticosteroids is not recommended. Patients with underlying respiratory conditions, such as acute exacerbation of asthma or chronic obstructive pulmonary disease (COPD), should receive steroids as indicated. Routine treatment with antibiotics is not indicated unless a bacterial superinfection is suspected or confirmed.

Table 1.1 Risk factors for severe disease [11]

Cancer
Cerebrovascular disease
Children with certain underlying conditions (such as asthma, developmental delay, congenital heart disease, and sickle cell disease)
Chronic kidney disease
COPD and other lung diseases (including interstitial lung disease, pulmonary fibrosis, pulmonary hypertension, cystic fibrosis)
Diabetes mellitus
Down syndrome
Cardiac conditions (e.g., heart failure, coronary artery disease, cardiomyopathies)
HIV infection
Neurologic conditions, including dementia
Obesity (BMI >30 kg/m2) and overweight (BMI 25 to 29 kg/m2)
Pregnancy
Smoking (current and former)
Sickle cell disease or thalassemia
Solid organ or blood stem cell transplantation
Substance use disorders
Use of corticosteroids or other immunosuppressive medications

It is advised against initiating anticoagulation or antiplatelet therapy in the outpatient setting.

Symptoms of COVID-19 can mimic many other common conditions; hence a broad differential diagnosis is important and should be investigated accordingly. The patient's existing medication regimen does not need to be adjusted. However, use of nebulized medications is preferably avoided to avoid transmission to other healthcare workers and patients. All patients are counseled on the warning symptoms that a clinician should promptly evaluate. All patients should be encouraged to provide a current healthcare proxy and advance directives.

On follow-up, the patient's respiratory status should be evaluated with the same criteria as that used for initial triage. Most patients discharged from the inpatient setting should have a follow-up visit within 2 days either by a teleconference or in-person clinic visit. Temporary housing in structured residential care facilities may be appropriate for some patients following their discharge from hospital.

1.10 Management of Hospitalized Adult Patients with Acute COVID-19

Indications for hospitalization and identification of patients who can be managed in the outpatient setting have been outlined in the beginning of this section.

Evaluation—The evaluation of hospitalized patients with documented COVID-19 should include assessing for risk factors associated with severe illness and identifying organ dysfunction or other comorbidities that could complicate therapy.

- Thromboprophylaxis—COVID-19 has a known association with thromboembolic complications; hence all patients hospitalized with moderate-severe disease should receive pharmacologic prophylaxis for venous thromboembolism as per local guidelines. It is yet unclear whether patients should receive thromboprophylaxis after discharge, and if so, for what duration? Decisions in this regard should be made on a case-by-case basis, primarily depending on risk of subsequent thrombosis.
- Antipyretics—Acetaminophen is widely used for fever management in patients with COVID-19. Guidelines do not recommend the use of nonsteroidal anti-inflammatory drugs (NSAIDs). If NSAIDs are required, then the lowest effective dose should be used. However, NSAIDs should not be discontinued in patients who were already using them for other conditions [12].
- Continuing chronic medications—Patients who are on an ACE inhibitor or ARB, should not stop their medication. Statins as well as aspirin may be continued in hospitalized patients with COVID-19 who are already taking them unless there is a specific concern of bleeding.

In patients with moderate disease, the care is primarily supportive, with close monitoring for disease progression. Additionally, patients with mild to moderate COVID-19 who are hospitalized for reasons other than COVID-19 may be evaluated and considered for monoclonal antibody therapy based on appropriate eligibility criteria.

- Approach to severe disease—For patients with severe disease (O_2 saturation $\leq$ 94% on room air or need for oxygenation or ventilatory support), COVID-19 therapy depends on the level of oxygen requirements and ordinal scale [13].
- For hospitalized patients with hypoxemia who are not yet on oxygen, intravenous remdesivir may be used. However, steroid use in these patients is discouraged.
- For hospitalized patients who are on low-flow supplemental oxygen, it is recommended to use low-dose steroids (dexamethasone/methylprednisolone) and IV remdesivir for 5 days. In patients with significantly elevated inflammatory markers and increasing oxygen requirements despite steroids, either baricitinib or tocilizumab may be added on a case-by-case basis.
- For hospitalized patients on high-flow supplemental oxygen or noninvasive ventilation, low dose dexamethasone should be used. For those who are admitted to an intensive care unit (ICU), either baricitinib or tocilizumab may be used in addition to steroids. The use of IV remdesivir may be extended to 10 days in such cases.

In hospitalized patients with severe disease who require mechanical ventilation or extracorporeal membrane oxygenation, low-dose steroids are recommended. Tocilizumab may be added especially in situations progressing to “cytokine storm.”

The use of other off-label drugs/therapies for the treatment of COVID-19 for hospitalized patients such as hydroxychloroquine, chloroquine, lopinavir-ritonavir, ivermectin, or convalescent plasma is not currently recommended.

1.11 Prognosis of Severe Disease

The mortality from COVID-19 appears driven primarily by the presence of severe ARDS. Several retrospective studies have reported variable mortality from COVID-19-related acute respiratory distress syndrome (ARDS), from 12 to 78%, with an average of 25 to 50%.

Mortality may be on the higher end of this range in resource-limited settings. Reducing mortality may reflect a younger patient population with a lower comorbidity burden during the subsequent surge, reduced burden on institutions, and/or growing expertise with COVID-19 care.

Prolonged symptoms are common during recovery from critical illness due to COVID-19, and many patients suffer from post-acute COVID-19 syndrome (PACS) [14]. In our experience, the rate of long-term complications in critically ill patients with COVID-19 may be higher than usual due to the prolonged nature of intubation and higher use of neuromuscular blockade and sedatives, with or without concurrent glucocorticoid administration. Long-term sequelae that can be seen in patients with COVID-19 and evaluation for and management of PACS are discussed separately.

References

1. SARS-CoV-2 variants of concern and variants under investigation in England. Technical briefing 31. December 10, 2021. https://assets.publishing.service.gov.uk/government/uploads/system/uploads/attachment_data/file/1040076/Technical_Briefing_31.pdf. Accessed on December 13, 2021.
2. SARS-CoV-2 variants of concern and variants under investigation. 33.
3. Li D, Jin M, Bao P, Zhao W, Zhang S. Clinical characteristics and results of semen tests among men with coronavirus disease 2019. JAMA Netw Open. 2020;3:e208292.
4. CDC. Quarantine & isolation [Internet]. Centers for disease control and prevention 2022 [cited 2022 Apr 15]; Available from: https://www.cdc.gov/coronavirus/2019-ncov/your-health/quarantine-isolation.html
5. Ma Q, Liu J, Liu Q, Kang L, Liu R, Jing W, et al. Global percentage of asymptomatic SARS-CoV-2 infections among the tested population and individuals with confirmed COVID-19 diagnosis: a systematic review and meta-analysis. JAMA Netw Open. 2021;4:e2137257.
6. CDC. Healthcare Workers [Internet]. Centers for disease control and prevention 2020 [cited 2022 Apr 15]; Available from: https://www.cdc.gov/coronavirus/2019-ncov/hcp/clinical-guidance-management-patients.html
7. Clinical features of covid-19 | The BMJ [Internet]. [cited 2022 Apr 15]; Available from: https://www.bmj.com/content/369/bmj.m1470/rapid-responses
8. Serum troponin, D-dimer, and CRP level in severe coronavirus (COVID-19) patients–PubMed [Internet]. [cited 2022 Apr 15]; Available from: https://pubmed.ncbi.nlm.nih.gov/34939346/

9. Dinnes J, Deeks JJ, Adriano A, Berhane S, Davenport C, Dittrich S, et al. Rapid, point-of-care antigen and molecular-based tests for diagnosis of SARS-CoV-2 infection. Cochrane Database Syst Rev. 2020;8:CD013705.
10. Early Treatment for Covid-19 with SARS-CoV-2 Neutralizing Antibody Sotrovimab | NEJM [Internet]. [cited 2022 Apr 15]; Available from: https://www.nejm.org/doi/full/10.1056/NEJMoa2107934
11. CDC. Cases, Data, and Surveillance [Internet]. Centers for Disease Control and Prevention 2020 [cited 2022 May 25]; Available from: https://www.cdc.gov/coronavirus/2019-ncov/covid-data/investigations-discovery/assessing-risk-factors.html
12. Concomitant Medications [Internet]. COVID-19 Treatment Guidelines [cited 2022 Apr 20]; Available from: https://www.covid19treatmentguidelines.nih.gov/therapies/concomitant-medications/
13. Marshall JC, Murthy S, Diaz J, Adhikari NK, Angus DC, Arabi YM, et al. A minimal common outcome measure set for COVID-19 clinical research. Lancet Infect Dis. 2020;20:e192–7.
14. Nalbandian A, Sehgal K, Gupta A, Madhavan MV, McGroder C, Stevens JS, et al. Post-acute COVID-19 syndrome. Nat Med. 2021;27:601–15.

Pulmonary Sequelae of COVID-19

2

Zubair Hasan, Abhinav Agrawal, and Mangala Narasimhan

2.1 Introduction

COVID-19 has affected over 280 million people globally, with over 240 million survivors. While the acute effects of COVID-19 are well understood, we are just beginning to understand the long-term effects of COVID-19, particularly as they relate to lung function and recovery. Persistent symptoms have been described as the post-acute sequelae of COVID-19 (PASC) and include short-term and long-term sequelae. Post-COVID-19 conditions can occur in patients who have had varying severity of illness during their acute infection. These include people who have had mild or even asymptomatic infections [1]. Post-COVID-19 conditions are referred to by a wide range of names, including long COVID, post-acute COVID-19, long-term effects of COVID-19, post-acute COVID syndrome, chronic COVID, long-haul COVID, and late sequelae, among others. Although standardized case definitions are still being developed, post-COVID-19 conditions can be considered a lack of return to a usual state of health following acute COVID-19 illness. The time frame for a post-COVID-19 condition is generally considered as 2–4 weeks following acute COVID-19 infection with incomplete resolution of symptoms or the emergence of new symptoms. Post-acute COVID-19 can be a multisystem condition. Around 10–35% of patients who have acute COVID-19 infection go on to develop long COVID symptoms [2]. The most common non-resolving symptoms are dyspnea, fatigue, malaise, cognitive impairment, cough, chest pain, palpitations, arthralgias, diarrhea, sleep difficulties, fever, light-headedness, continued anosmia, and mood changes. For hospitalized patients, the incidence of the post-COVID-19 syndrome may reach as high as 85% [2]. Post-COVID-19 sequelae can be highly

Z. Hasan · A. Agrawal · M. Narasimhan (✉)
Donald and Barbara Zucker School of Medicine at Hofstra/Northwell, Hempstead, NY, USA

A. Mohan, S. Mittal (eds.), *Post COVID-19 Complications and Management*,
https://doi.org/10.1007/978-981-19-4407-9_2

debilitating and seriously impact occupational and social activities. It also will add significantly to the healthcare burden in addition to its consequences on mental health.

2.2 Pathophysiology

There are several proposed mechanisms for long COVID. One theory proposes that SARS-CoV-2 viral persistence in the body contributes to immune activation and long COVID symptoms. The evidence for this is an increased level of inflammatory biomarkers such as C-reactive protein (CRP), interleukin-6 (IL-6), and D-dimer in patients with long COVID [3]. Another proposed mechanism suggests that cell dysfunction promotes long COVID pathophysiology similar to an autoimmune disorder [4]. There have been autopsy reports of infiltrates in the lungs and other organs that are CD8+ T cell-enriched, which would be evidence of an ongoing autoimmune reaction [5]. There is also evidence that severe COVID-19 causes lymphopenia with both B and T cell deficiency. This causes hyperinflammation as T cells participate in inflammation resolution. Serum samples from COVID-19 patients show an increased incidence of antiphospholipid autoantibodies which is associated with more severe clinical outcomes [6]. However, it is still not completely clear which of these mechanisms is dominant, or whether combinations of mechanisms cause long COVID.

2.3 Respiratory Clinical Features of Post-Acute Sequelae of COVID-19

Patients with acute COVID-19 are expected to have symptoms for up to 4 weeks following an initial illness. Those patients with ongoing symptoms beyond 2 months after their initial COVID-19 illness are considered to have post-acute sequelae of SARS-CoV-2, otherwise known as long COVID [7]. These symptoms vary widely and can include neurocognitive and physical symptoms, many of them respiratory in nature. Based on several published reports, the table below shows the approximate proportion of clinical respiratory symptoms of long COVID. However, this information is evolving as new data emerges (Table 2.1).

Table 2.1 Percentage of patients with respiratory clinical features of long COVID

Long COVID respiratory symptom	Percentage of patients affected
Dyspnea	16 to 66% [8–12]
Chest discomfort	8 to 44% [9–12]
Cough	7 to 34% [10–12]
Fatigue	31 to 72% [8–12]
Throat pain	3% [10]
Sputum production	3% [10]

2.4 Radiological Abnormalities

Many reports have found radiological evidence of lung fibrosis that can last up to 6 months after initial hospital discharge from COVID-19 pneumonia [13, 14]. In a 3-month follow-up study of COVID-19 survivors, pulmonary radiological abnormalities were detected in 71% of patients, and functional impairments were detected in 25% of participants. Only 10% of patients in this study had severe pneumonia when diagnosed initially with COVID-19 [15]. Another study observed reduced lung diffusion capacity that correlated with radiological abnormalities in 42% of COVID-19 survivors at 3 months posthospital discharge, regardless of initial disease severity [16]. Even 6 months after symptom onset, lung radiological abnormalities associated with persistent symptoms were still present in about half of COVID-19 survivors [17]. There is evidence of chronic scar formation in the lungs that may be responsible for persistent dyspnea and cough. This scarring may not always be visible on a CT scan but indirectly suggested by a reduction in diffusion capacity [18]. In addition, another study of COVID-19 survivors with persistent symptoms after 4 weeks showed persistent inflammation via increased FDG uptake in the bone marrow and blood vessels [19].

2.5 Pulmonary Function Testing

While the COVID-19 pandemic is still ongoing and long-term data is limited, there is some prior experience in similar diseases for clinicians to better understand what to expect with post-COVID-19 patients, especially those who develop acute respiratory distress syndrome (ARDS). Patients who develop ARDS are known to have long-term pulmonary sequelae. In a study of 78 patients with ARDS, 80% had persistent reduction in $D_{L_{CO}}$ on pulmonary function tests (PFTs) 1 year post-hospitalization [20]. Twenty percent had a restrictive lung disease pattern, and 20% had obstructive lung disease patterns, although most of these patients were smokers at the time of their infection [14]. This held true regardless of the ventilation strategy the patient underwent during their ARDS, either low or high tidal volume ventilation. This is particularly relevant to COVID-19 patients given the heterogeneity in lung compliance and ventilation strategies [21]. In addition to PFT abnormalities, patients are known to have abnormalities on imaging that persist even 1 year post-ARDS, particularly related to signs of pulmonary fibrosis [14] (Fig. 2.1).

The influenza A (H1N1 subtype) pandemic in 2009 gives us some guidance on what we may come to expect with patients recovering from COVID-19. During the H1N1 pandemic, the US Centers for Disease Control and Prevention (CDC) estimated that there were over 60 million cases in the United States, of which over 270,000 were hospitalized and over 12,000 died. Patients with H1N1 typically developed pneumonia-like symptoms of hypoxemia, with many developing ARDS. In a study of nine patients with H1N1-related ARDS, six had at least a mild reduction in FEV1, and five of the nine had at least a mild reduction of FVC 1 month

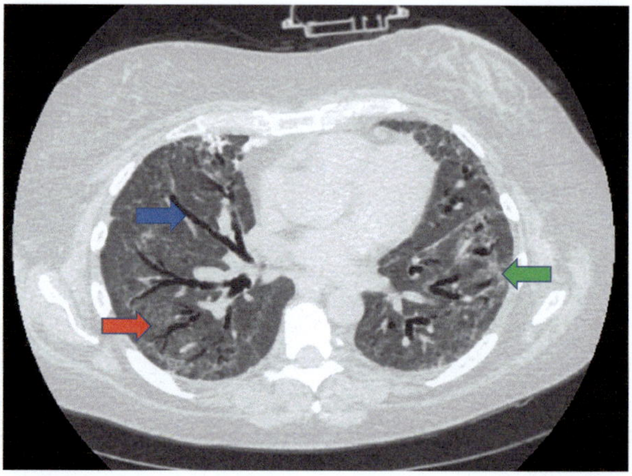

Fig. 2.1 CT chest features of post-covid pulmonary abnormalities. This CT shows traction bronchiectasis (blue arrow) and reticular markings (red arrow) in a background of ground glass opacities (green arrow)

after discharge from their hospitalization [22]. At 6 months post-discharge, all patients had normalized FEV1, and most had normalized FVC. Total lung capacity (TLC) was reduced in six patients at 1 month, with only two patients regaining normal TLC by 6 months. DLCO was low in seven of nine patients at 1 month and remained persistently low in four of the nine patients at 6 months. Almost all patients had reduced six-minute walk distances (6MWD) based on their predicted values at 1 month post-discharge, with improvement to normal at 3 months. Of note, all these patients were enrolled in pulmonary rehabilitation programs. This study, therefore, showed that all patients with H1N1-related ARDS developed some pulmonary function abnormalities. While most of them had largely recovered, some continued to have persistent abnormalities, especially reduced diffusion even at 6 months post-discharge.

Patients with mild influenza developed longer-term PFT abnormalities as well. In another study of 48 patients with mild H1N1, 33% had a persistent reduction in DLCO 1 year post-discharge, along with 33% with evidence of small airway disease, as evidenced by decreased forced expiratory flow at 50% and 75% of forced vital capacity [23]. Many patients had evidence of restrictive lung disease that persisted for 1 year post-discharge, though whether this was merely due to unmasking of underlying lung disease pre-H1N1 is unclear as most of these patients did not have a prior spirometry.

Another correlate for the current pandemic is based on the literature from the severe acute respiratory syndrome (SARS) pandemic in 2003, which was also caused by a coronavirus. One study found that one-third of SARS survivors had impairments in pulmonary function 1 year post-discharge, with the most common abnormalities seen in the FEV1 and DLCO [24]. There was no significant difference between patients with varying disease severity 1 year post-discharge, although the patients with decreased DLCO were more likely to have fibrosis on imaging.

In summary, previous literature has shown that patients who become hospitalized with ARDS are known to have abnormal pulmonary function tests up to 1 year post-discharge, marked by restrictive lung disease patterns and reduced DLCO. Some patients who had H1N1 or SARS had abnormal PFTs at least 1 year post-discharge, though the improvement was noted in those who underwent pulmonary rehabilitation. This is critical to understand as it informs our ongoing management of patients with post-acute sequelae of COVID-19.

2.6 Current Understanding of Lung Function Tests in Patients with COVID-19

While PFTs are integral to objectively determine the actual effect of COVID-19 on the lungs, given the concern of how the virus is transmitted, pulmonary function laboratories have been cautious about restarting testing. Many of the patients from early in the COVID-19 pandemic are just starting to have meaningful pulmonary function follow-up almost 2 years after their initial diagnoses. As a result, we are just starting to understand the longer-term implications of COVID-19 infection on pulmonary function.

Of patients admitted early in the pandemic, many now display restrictive patterns of lung disease like other viral pneumonia and ARDS patients in the past. In an Italian study of patients with COVID-19 early in the pandemic, FEV1 and FVC were all lower than their lower limit of normal values and only started to improve after 6 weeks post-discharge [25]. However, these were patients that were sick enough to require hospital admission, and results were available based on a short-term follow-up only. The restrictive pattern seen on these PFTs mirrors the pattern seen after long-term follow-up of past respiratory diseases like influenza and SARS.

It is less clear if the severity of the initial COVID-19 illness has a bearing on pulmonary function over a long period of time. Most studies to date have broken down COVID-19 disease by those with mild symptoms (no clinical pneumonia), moderate disease (clinical pneumonia but no significant hypoxemia), and severe disease (RR > 30, SpO2 < 94% on room air). In a study of 57 patients, of which 70% had non-severe COVID-19 and completed PFTs at least 2 weeks post-discharge, the group means for FEV1, FVC, and FEV1/FVC ratio were within normal limits, with no statistically significant difference between disease severity in these parameters [26]. However, many patients had abnormal values in each of these domains. Patients with severe disease did have a more significant decline in total lung capacity compared to non-severe disease. About 52.6% had abnormal diffusion capacity, with a higher impairment rate in patients with severe disease. Similarly, patients with severe disease had a significantly shorter 6MWD than those with non-severe disease, both in absolute distance and % predicted, with severe cases achieving 88% predicted 6MWD. While none of the patients in the study had a chronic respiratory disease, over a third had a prior medical illness, including hypertension, and nine patients had a smoking history, all of which may play a role in their persistent PFT abnormalities [20].

A larger systematic review including 380 patients post-COVID-19 showed that 15% of patients had a restrictive pattern on spirometry, 7% had an obstructive pattern, and 39% had impaired DLCO [27]. The prevalence of impaired DLCO was greatest in those with severe COVID-19. However, some patients had pulmonary function testing done 1 month after the onset of symptoms or 1 to 3 months post-discharge, which may skew the results, as some of the abnormalities may just be due to the acute phase of the disease. This mirrors another systematic review of 57 studies, including over 250,000 survivors of COVID-19 who were assessed for PASC at least 1 month after COVID-19 infection [28]. In this review, 65% of patients had increased oxygen requirements, 30.3% had diffusion abnormalities, and 10% had restrictive lung disease on spirometry.

Patients with pulmonary function test abnormalities after COVID-19 are also more likely to have radiographic abnormalities that persist months after their initial diagnosis. As many as 55% of patients in one study had some radiographic abnormality after a mean follow-up of approximately 12 weeks after their COVID-19 diagnosis [29]. Of this group, 85% had ground-glass opacities, and 65% had reticulation on imaging, suggesting developing fibrosis from the profound inflammatory response from ARDS due to COVID-19.

Together, these studies suggest that patients with COVID-19 are likely to develop at least short-term pulmonary function test abnormalities showing restrictive lung disease and impaired diffusion, with a smaller subset developing obstructive lung disease. Most patients with mild and moderate COVID-19 disease will recover some degree of their FEV1, FVC, and TLC, though as disease severity worsens, patients are more likely to have persistent impairments in DLCO. Further long-term data is needed to assess the long-term effect of COVID-19 on pulmonary function truly. In addition, the impact of pulmonary rehabilitation on improving lung function akin to its effect on other viral syndrome-associated ARDS also needs to be studied.

2.7 Illustrative Case

A 55-year-old smoker male had required hospitalization and supplemental oxygen due to severe COVID-19 pneumonia. His CT thorax done 2 months following discharge demonstrates bilateral peripheral linear opacities and ground-glass opacities (Fig. 2.2). His pulmonary function testing was done 3 months post-COVID-19 infection and was suggestive of restrictive lung disease with a decreased FEV1 compared to the lower limit of normal (LLN) and decreased diffusion capacity (DLCO) (Figs. 2.3 and 2.4).

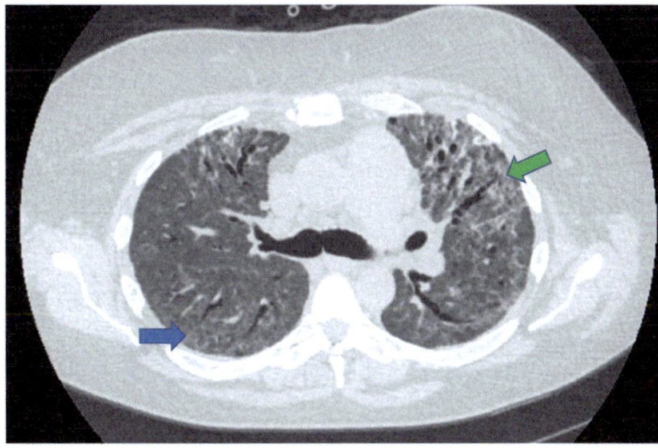

Fig. 2.2 CT chest of illustrative case. This CT shows peripheral linear opacities (blue arrow) and ground glass opacities (green arrow)

		Ref	LLN-ULN	Pre	% Ref
Spirometry					
FVC	Liters	4.48	(3.6 - 5.3)	3.24	72
FEV1	Liters	3.44	(2.7 - 4.2)	2.54	74
FEV1/FVC	%	77	(67.0 - 86.4)	78	
FEV1/SVC	%			78	
FEF25-75%	L/sec	2.98	(1.5 - 4.5)	2.23	75
PEF	L/sec	8.97	(6.8 - 11.1)	10.27	115
FET100%	Sec			8.45	
FEF/FIF50				0.50	
Vol Extrap	Liters			0.02	

Fig. 2.3 Spirometry of Illustrative case

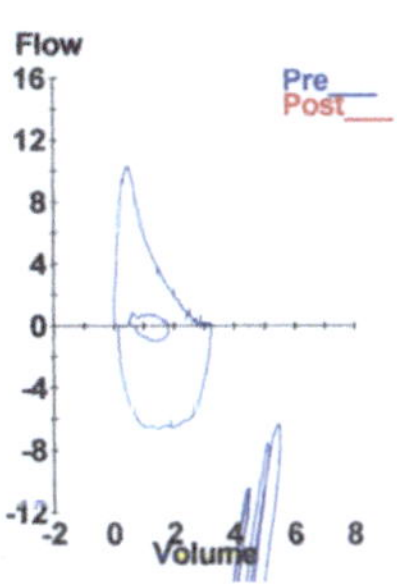

Lung Volumes					
TLC	Liters	6.47		4.65	72
VC	Liters	4.48	(3.6 - 5.3)	3.24	72
IC	Liters	3.20		1.94	61
FRC PL	Liters	3.28	(1.8 - 4.7)	2.71	83
ERV	Liters	1.28		1.23	96
RV	Liters	1.99	(1.2 - 2.8)	1.41	71
RV/TLC	%	31		30	
Vtg	Liters	3.41	(2.4 - 4.4)	3.81	112
Vtg f	BPM			100	
Diffusing Capacity					
DLCO	mL/min/mmHg	28.4	(20.5 - 36.4)	14.9	53
DL Adj	mL/min/mmHg	28.4	(20.5 - 36.4)	14.9	53
DL/VA Adj	mL/min/mHg/L	4.02	(2.2 - 5.9)	3.63	90
VA	Liters	6.47		4.12	64
IVC	Liters	3.24	(2.9 - 3.6)	3.04	94

Fig. 2.4 Diffusion capacity and lung volume measurements of illustrative case

2.8 Management of Post-COVID-19 Respiratory Sequelae

Patients who recover from the acute phase of COVID-19 may continue to have signs and symptoms of disease that persist at least 2 months after their initial illness, at which point they would be diagnosed with post-acute sequelae of COVID-19, or long COVID [30]. These symptoms are usually persistent cough, sore throat, fatigue, "brain fog," and dyspnea. Patients with chronic cough often seek antitussive therapies, but it is unknown whether these are effective in post-COVID-19 cough. In the clinical management of post-COVID-19 chronic cough, it is important to exclude any pathological or structural causes such as fibrotic damage to the lung parenchyma or damage to the airway caused by the acute illness and its treatment (e.g., endotracheal intubation-related complications). The classic evaluation for chronic cough should also be performed to exclude conditions such as gastroesophageal reflux disease, ACE inhibitor-induced cough, lung fibrosis, or airway inflammation [31]. A persistent cough in post-COVID-19 syndrome may be driven by neuroinflammation leading to a state of laryngeal and cough hypersensitivity. Gabapentin and pregabalin, which are neuromodulators, have been shown to be effective in controlling chronic refractory cough [32]. Inhaled steroids have been studied for a chronic cough from COVID-19, and have not been shown to be effective [33]. Management of cognitive impairment and fatigue is currently under evaluation and not yet established. The dyspnea needs a full work-up to evaluate for fibrosis, pulmonary embolism, and other classic causes of dyspnea. With research still ongoing, it is anticipated to have more clarity on effective symptom-based therapies in the future.

There is no universal consensus on how these patients with long COVID should be evaluated, but some societies have proposed guidelines. The British Thoracic Society recommends that patients with mild COVID-19 who are still symptomatic be followed up at 3 months for a clinical assessment and with a chest X-ray, with further work-up, such as PFTs, 6-minute walk tests, and echocardiograms based on clinical judgment [30]. Others suggest getting a chest X-ray, PFTs, and 6-minute walk tests at their initial visit to establish a baseline and then repeating them at three monthly intervals [34]. There is no consensus on the optimum timing for obtaining chest computed tomography (chest CT), though some suggest that it be done in patients with long COVID symptoms at their initial visit and then 6 and 12 months afterward.

Some patients develop ground-glass opacities (GGO) with subpleural and peribronchial consolidations suggestive of organizing pneumonia after having had COVID-19. Corticosteroids are the mainstay of treatment for organizing pneumonia. In a study of patients with persistent interstitial lung changes treated with steroids, many suggestive of organizing pneumonia, the vast majority had improvement in their dyspnea scores, FVC, DLCO, and 6MWT, as well as improvement in their radiographic abnormalities [35]. All patients had presumably cleared their virus based on the timeline of infection. This suggests that in patients with abnormal PFTs with persistent radiographic changes of ground-glass opacities or consolidations post-COVID-19 but no fibrosis or active infection, corticosteroids may be beneficial for improvement in dyspnea, PFT, and radiographic abnormalities. However, the optimum dose of steroids is not yet standardized. In one observational study of patients with persistent interstitial lung disease (predominantly organizing pneumonia at least 6 weeks after COVID-19 infection), patients received corticosteroids up to a maximum dose of 0.5 mg/kg of prednisolone and were tapered over 3 weeks. This led to an improvement in their functional status, as well as lung function based on PFTs [35]. Another open-label randomized trial of COVID-19 patients with persistent dyspnea, hypoxemia, or radiological abnormalities at least 3 weeks post-COVID-19 illness compared high-dose (prednisolone 40 mg/day tapered over 6 weeks) versus prednisolone 10 mg daily for 6 weeks [36]. Both groups benefited from corticosteroid treatment and demonstrated an improvement in radiological findings, spirometry, and dyspnea at 6 weeks. Most importantly, there was no significant difference in outcomes between the two groups, suggesting that even low-dose corticosteroids may benefit many patients [34].

It is also not clear how to manage patients with obvious fibrotic changes post-COVID-19. After the SARS outbreak in 2003, many patients developed pulmonary fibrosis on CT, with one study showing that 15/24 patients had fibrosis on CT scan at mean follow-up of 37 days post-discharge, with patients requiring ICU being more likely to develop fibrosis [37]. There are many postulated reasons as to why patients with ARDS develop pulmonary fibrosis, starting with the inflammatory phase of ARDS and its progression into the fibrotic phase. These include the dysregulated release of matrix metalloproteinases leading to fibroproliferation and vascular dysfunction leading to fibrosis, possibly due to VEGF, and cytokines such as IL-6 and TNF-α [38].

Since the cascade of events eventually leading to fibrosis starts very early on in ARDS, the role for anti-fibrotic therapies early in COVID-19-related ARDS has been considered and evaluated. Nintedanib can reduce bronchoalveolar lavage concentrations of IL-1, a known player in the pathogenesis of idiopathic pulmonary fibrosis, and pirfenidone reduces serum and lung IL-6 concentrations in mouse models of pulmonary fibrosis [26]. However, this is just a biological rationale for the novel treatment of COVID-19. Based on current evidence, it is still unclear if anti-fibrotic agents have any definite role preventing further fibrosis in patients who have recovered from their acute COVID-19 illness. In the INBUILD trial of nintedanib in patients with progressive pulmonary fibrosis due to various disorders, those who received nintedanib had a reduction in FVC decline and therefore benefited from treatment [35]. Given that some patients with progressive fibrotic lung diseases and even patients with COVID-19 have immune dysregulation as a shared pathogenetic mechanism, it has been hoped that early anti-fibrotic therapy may prevent or retard the development of COVID-19-associated fibrosis. As of now, however, there are no published long-term studies of these anti-fibrotic agents in post-COVID-19 respiratory syndromes, although several trials are ongoing.

Lastly, many patients with persistent dyspnea and impaired lung function post COVID-19 may benefit from pulmonary rehabilitation. In 1 observational cohort study, 50 patients with mild to severe COVID-19 and reduced 6MWD and impaired FVC at least 3 months after their initial diagnosis were enrolled in pulmonary rehabilitation. After 3 weeks of pulmonary rehabilitation, all patients demonstrated an improvement in their FVC and 6MWD, with patients with mild COVID-19 gaining a median of 48 meters and those with severe COVID-19 gaining 124 meters [39]. This implies that pulmonary rehabilitation should be an essential part of therapy for patients with respiratory post-acute sequelae of COVID-19.

2.9 Conclusion

Post-COVID-19 sequelae can have a serious impact on the ability to return to normal functional status. There can be significant economic and mental health consequences for the person with the illness, their families, and the communities they live in. Thus, a multidisciplinary and multispecialty approach is required for a holistic management of these patients. Some treatment algorithms include steroid therapy and pulmonary rehabilitation, and interval pulmonary testing. Educational materials to alert patients of symptoms and seek help post-acute infection should also be distributed. Another important aspect is the development of patient registries to support research efforts to understand and treat post-acute COVID-19 sequelae. As a pulmonary community, it seems that we will be dealing with post-COVID-19 syndromes for a long time.

References

1. Havervall S, Rosell A, Phillipson M, et al. Symptoms and functional impairment assessed 8 months after mild COVID-19 among health care workers. JAMA. 2021;325(19):2015–6. https://doi.org/10.1001/jama.2021.5612.
2. Pavli A, Theodoridou M, Maltezou HC. Post-COVID syndrome: incidence, clinical Spectrum, and challenges for primary healthcare professionals. Arch Med Res. 2021;6(52):575–81. SSN 0188-4409. https://doi.org/10.1016/j.arcmed.2021.03.010.
3. Marvisi M, Ferrozzi F, Balzarini L, et al. First report on clinical and radiological features of COVID-19 pneumonitis in a Caucasian population: factors predicting fibrotic evolution. Int J Infect Dis. 2020;99:485–8.
4. Karlsson AC, Humbert M, Buggert M. The known unknowns of T cell immunity to COVID. Sci Immunol. 2020;5(53):19.
5. Ehrenfeld M, Tincani A, Andreoli L, et al. Covid-19 and autoimmunity. Autoimmun Rev. 2020;19(8):102597.
6. Zuo Y, Estes SK, Ali RA, et al. Prothrombotic autoantibodies in serum from patients hospitalized with COVID-19. Sci Transl Med. 2020;12:eabd3876.
7. Soriano JB, Murthy S, Marshall JC, Relan P, Diaz JV, WHO Clinical Case Definition Working Group on Post-COVID-19 Condition. A clinical case definition of post-COVID-19 condition by a Delphi consensus. Lancet. Infectious diseases. 2021;S1473-3099(21):00703–9. https://doi.org/10.1016/S1473-3099(21)00703-9.
8. Halpin SJ, McIvor C, Whyatt G, Adams A, Harvey O, McLean L, Walshaw C, Kemp S, Corrado J, Singh R, Collins T, O'Connor RJ, Sivan M. Postdischarge symptoms and rehabilitation needs in survivors of COVID-19 infection: a cross-sectional evaluation. J Med Virol. 2021;93(2):1013–22. https://doi.org/10.1002/jmv.26368.
9. Writing Committee for the COMEBAC Study Group, Morin L, Savale L, Pham T, Colle R, Figueiredo S, Harrois A, Gasnier M, Lecoq AL, Meyrignac O, Noel N, Baudry E, Bellin

MF, Beurnier A, Choucha W, Corruble E, Dortet L, Hardy-Leger I, Radiguer F, Sportouch S, et al. Four-month clinical status of a cohort of patients after hospitalization for COVID-19. JAMA. 2021;325(15):1525–34. https://doi.org/10.1001/jama.2021.3331.
10. Xiong Q, Xu M, Li J, Liu Y, Zhang J, Xu Y, Dong W. Clinical sequelae of COVID-19 survivors in Wuhan, China: a single-Centre longitudinal study. Clin Microbiol Infect. 2021;27(1):89–95. https://doi.org/10.1016/j.cmi.2020.09.023.
11. Carfì A, Bernabei R, Landi F, Gemelli Against COVID-19 Post-Acute Care Study Group. Persistent symptoms in patients after acute COVID-19. JAMA. 2020;324(6):603–5. https://doi.org/10.1001/jama.2020.12603.
12. Cares-Marambio K, Montenegro-Jiménez Y, Torres-Castro R, Vera-Uribe R, Torralba Y, Alsina-Restoy X, Vasconcello-Castillo L, Vilaró J. Prevalence of potential respiratory symptoms in survivors of hospital admission after coronavirus disease 2019 (COVID-19): a systematic review and meta-analysis. Chron Respir Dis. 2021;18:14799731211002240. https://doi.org/10.1177/14799731211002240.
13. Bellan M, Soddu D, Balbo PE, et al. Respiratory and psychophysical sequelae among patients with COVID-19 four months after hospital discharge. JAMA Netw Open. 2021;4(1):e2036142.
14. Han X, Fan Y, Alwalid O, et al. Six-month follow-up chest CT findings after severe COVID-19 pneumonia. Radiology. 2021;299(1):E177–86.
15. Zhao YM, Shang YM, Song WB, et al. Follow-up study of the pulmonary function and related physiological characteristics of COVID-19 survivors three months after recovery. E Clin Med. 2020;25:100463.
16. van den Borst B, et al. Comprehensive health assessment three months after recovery from acute COVID-19. Clin Infect Dis 2020;ciaa1750.
17. Huang C, Huang L, Wang Y, et al. 6-month consequences of COVID-19 in patients discharged from hospital: a cohort study. Lancet. 2021;397(10270):220–32.
18. Swigris JJ, Streiner DL, Brown KK, et al. Assessing exertional dyspnea in patients with idiopathic pulmonary fibrosis. Respir Med. 2014;108(1):181–8.
19. Sollini M, et al. Vasculitis changes in COVID-19 survivors with persistent symptoms: an [(18) F]FDG-PET/CT study. Eur J Nucl Med Mol Imaging. 2020;48(5):1460–6.
20. Orme J Jr, Romney JS, Hopkins RO, Pope D, Chan KJ, Thomsen G, Crapo RO, Weaver LK. Pulmonary function and health-related quality of life in survivors of acute respiratory distress syndrome. Am J Respir Crit Care Med. 2003;167(5):690–4.
21. Marini JJ, Gattinoni L. Management of COVID-19 respiratory distress. JAMA. 2020;323(22):2329–30.
22. Hsieh MJ, Lee WC, Cho HY, Wu MF, Hu HC, Kao KC, Chen NH, Tsai YH, Huang CC. Recovery of pulmonary functions, exercise capacity, and quality of life after pulmonary rehabilitation in survivors of ARDS due to severe influenza a (H1N1) pneumonitis. Influenza Other Respir Viruses. 2018;12(5):643–8.
23. Liu W, Peng L, Liu H, Hua S. Pulmonary function and clinical manifestations of patients infected with mild influenza a virus subtype H1N1: a one-year follow-up. PLoS One. 2015;10(7):e0133698.
24. Ong KC, Ng AW, Lee LS, Kaw G, Kwek SK, Leow MK, Earnest A. 1-year pulmonary function and health status in survivors of severe acute respiratory syndrome. Chest. 2005;128(3):1393–400.
25. Fumagalli A, Misuraca C, Bianchi A, Borsa N, Limonta S, Maggiolini S, Bonardi DR, Corsonello A, Di Rosa M, Soraci L, Lattanzio F, Colombo D. Pulmonary function in patients surviving to COVID-19 pneumonia. Infection. 2021;49(1):153–7.
26. Huang Y, Tan C, Wu J, Chen M, Wang Z, Luo L, Zhou X, Liu X, Huang X, Yuan S, Chen C, Gao F, Huang J, Shan H, Liu J. Impact of coronavirus disease 2019 on pulmonary function in early convalescence phase. Respir Res. 2020;21(1):163.
27. Torres-Castro R, Vasconcello-Castillo L, Alsina-Restoy X, Solis-Navarro L, Burgos F, Puppo H, Vilaró J. Respiratory function in patients post-infection by COVID-19: a systematic review and meta analysis. Pulmonology. 2021;27(4):328–37.

28. Groff D, Sun A, Ssentongo AE, Ba DM, Parsons N, Poudel GR, Lekoubou A, Oh JS, Ericson JE, Ssentongo P, Chinchilli VM. Short-term and long-term rates of Postacute sequelae of SARS-CoV-2 infection: a systematic review. JAMA Netw Open. 2021;4(10):e2128568.
29. Shah AS, Wong AW, Hague CJ, Murphy DT, Johnston JC, Ryerson CJ, Carlsten C. A prospective study of 12-week respiratory outcomes in COVID-19-related hospitalisations. Thorax. 2021;76(4):402–4.
30. Nalbandian A, Sehgal K, Gupta A, Madhavan MV, McGroder C, Stevens JS, Cook JR, Nordvig AS, Shalev D, Sehrawat TS, Ahluwalia N, Bikdeli B, Dietz D, Der-Nigoghossian C, Liyanage-Don N, Rosner GF, Bernstein EJ, Mohan S, Beckley AA, Seres DS, et al. Post-acute COVID-19 syndrome. Nat Med. 2021;27(4):601–15. https://doi.org/10.1038/s41591-021-01283-z.
31. Gibson P, Wang G, McGarvey L, et al. Treatment of unexplained chronic cough: CHEST guideline and expert panel report. Chest. 2016;149:27–44.
32. Ryan NM, Birring SS, Gibson PG. Gabapentin for refractory chronic cough: a randomised, double-blind, placebo-controlled trial. Lancet. 2012;380:1583–9.
33. Clemency BM, Varughese R, Gonzalez-Rojas Y, et al. Efficacy of inhaled Ciclesonide for outpatient treatment of adolescents and adults with symptomatic COVID-19: a randomized clinical trial. JAMA Intern Med. 2022;182(1):42–9. https://doi.org/10.1001/jamainternmed.2021.6759.
34. Raghu G, Wilson KC. COVID-19 interstitial pneumonia: monitoring the clinical course in survivors. Lancet Respir Med. 2020;8(9):839–42. https://doi.org/10.1016/S2213-2600(20)30349-0.
35. Myall KJ, Mukherjee B, Castanheira AM, Lam JL, Benedetti G, Mak SM, Preston R, Thillai M, Dewar A, Molyneaux PL, West AG. Persistent post-COVID-19 interstitial lung disease. An observational study of corticosteroid treatment. Ann Am Thorac Soc. 2021;18(5):799–806.
36. Dhooria S, Chaudhary S, Sehgal IS, Agarwal R, Arora S, Garg M, Prabhakar N, Puri GD, Bhalla A, Suri V, Yaddanapudi LN, Muthu V, Prasad KT, Aggarwal AN. High-dose versus low-dose prednisolone in symptomatic patients with post-COVID-19 diffuse parenchymal lung abnormalities: an open-label, randomised trial (acronym: COLDSTER). Eur Respir J. 2021;2102930. Advance online publication https://doi.org/10.1183/13993003.02930-2021.
37. Antonio GE, Wong KT, Hui DS, Wu A, Lee N, Yuen EH, Leung CB, Rainer TH, Cameron P, Chung SS, Sung JJ, Ahuja AT. Thin-section CT in patients with severe acute respiratory syndrome following hospital discharge: preliminary experience. Radiology. 2003;228(3):810–5.
38. George PM, Wells AU, Jenkins RG. Pulmonary fibrosis and COVID-19: the potential role for antifibrotic therapy. Lancet Respir Med. 2020;8(8):807–15.
39. Gloeckl R, Leitl D, Jarosch I, Schneeberger T, Nell C, Stenzel N, Vogelmeier CF, Kenn K, Koczulla AR. Benefits of pulmonary rehabilitation in COVID-19: a prospective observational cohort study. ERJ Open Res. 2021;7(2):00108–2021. https://doi.org/10.1183/23120541.00108-2021.

Role of Imaging in Post-COVID-19 Complications

3

Ashu Seith Bhalla, Priyanka Naranje, and Abhishek Jayant

As the COVID-19 pandemic continues to rage across the world with a waxing and waning course, the number of patients with long COVID (more than 4 weeks) and post-COVID-19 (more than 12 weeks) conditions continues to grow. Since the lung is the dominantly affected organ, the majority of the symptomatic sequelae also pertain to the respiratory system. Among others, pulmonary fibrosis is recognized as an important type of post-acute sequelae of COVID-19 (PASC) [1, 2].

As imaging is a primary part of the initial diagnosis of COVID-19 pneumonia, it remains a key component of follow-up assessment, particularly in those patients with moderate or severe disease. This chapter focuses on the imaging of patients with suspected post-COVID-19 pulmonary sequelae.

3.1 Imaging Modalities

The primary imaging modalities for evaluation of post-COVID-19 patients include chest radiograph, computed tomography (CT) of the thorax, and CT pulmonary angiogram. Ultrasound of the lung has also been used to assess patients for post-COVID-19 sequelae; however, its utility is not yet clearly defined. The British Thoracic Society has published guidance about the respiratory follow-up of patients with COVID-19 pneumonia [3]. The recommendations divided patients into two groups: those with a severe disease with or without ICU admissions and those with mild to moderate disease managed in the ward or community. In both situations, the first follow-up imaging is recommended at 12 weeks and is a chest radiograph/chest X-ray (CXR). Subsequent decision to do a computed tomogram (CT) and the type

A. S. Bhalla (✉) · P. Naranje · A. Jayant
Department of Radiodiagnosis and Interventional Radiology, All India Institute of Medical Sciences, New Delhi, India

A. Mohan, S. Mittal (eds.), *Post COVID-19 Complications and Management*, https://doi.org/10.1007/978-981-19-4407-9_3

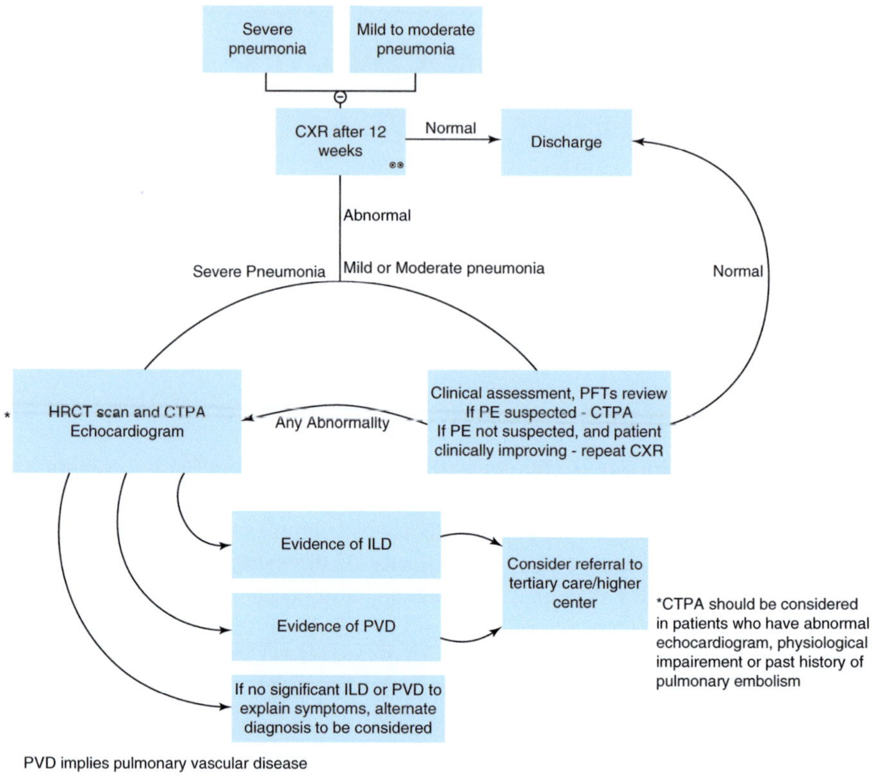

Fig. 3.1 Modified algorithm for follow-up of patients of COVID-19 pneumonia

of CT (high-resolution CT [HRCT] or CT pulmonary angiography [CTPA]) is based on CXR findings and initial disease severity or presence of persistent respiratory symptoms. Based on these guidelines, a suggested algorithm for follow-up of patients with COVID-19 pneumonia is given in Fig. 3.1, and an illustrative case is shown in Fig. 3.2.

However, there is an ongoing debate whether CXRs should be performed at all, and several authors recommend performing CT scans as the initial imaging modality, as CXR may miss or underestimate pulmonary changes [1]. A reasonable approach would be to perform a CT scan in those with persistent breathlessness, even if CXR is normal. If patients are started on therapy using steroids or antifibrotics, CXRs are helpful as detailed above for initial screening and intermittent follow-up, particularly in those with minimal/mild symptoms. However, CT thorax is needed for detailed response evaluation.

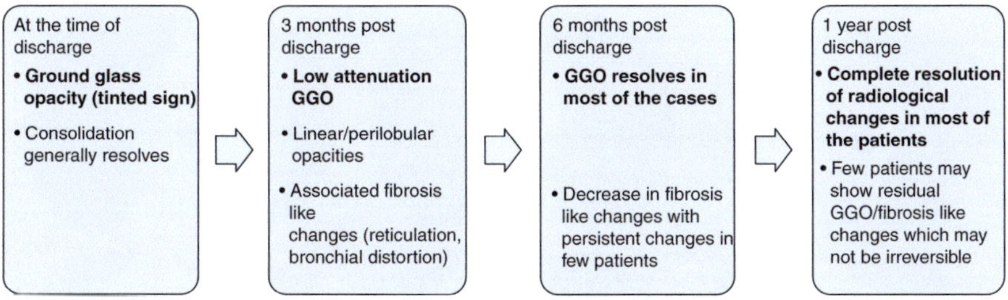

Fig. 3.2 Evolution of imaging findings on CT over time in COVID-19 pneumonia

3.2 Imaging Findings

Based on the stages of COVID-19 pneumonia, its initial severity, and time elapsed since the initial infection, various combinations of imaging findings of ground-glass opacities (GGOs), consolidations, reticular opacities, and bronchial dilatation are seen. Literature is now available on serial imaging findings in patients following COVID-19 pneumonia. Collating these findings, the evolution of changes is better understood (Fig. 3.3) [4, 5]. Further, a recent proposition paper elucidates the *glossary of terms* to be employed while reporting post-COVID-19 imaging studies [6].

3.2.1 Ground-Glass Opacity (GGO)

Ground-glass opacities (GGOs) are the signature of COVID-19 pneumonia in the acute phase. In general, the presence of GGOs on imaging can be the consequence of several pathophysiologic phenomena such as alveolar filling, interstitial edema, or mosaic perfusion. When superimposed with septal thickening, or bronchial dilatation, it could represent an area of early fibrosis.

In the context of COVID-19 pneumonia, as pneumonia resolves, the density of the GGO reduces, resulting in *low-density GGO*. Occasionally the reduction in GGO density may be accompanied by a paradoxical increase in the area involved; this may be misinterpreted as deterioration and is referred to as a “tinted sign” [6] (Fig. 3.4).

3.2.2 Consolidation

Consolidation can be seen in acute COVID-19 pneumonia, particularly in moderate and severe disease. In severe disease, the diffuse alveolar damage/ARDS development is associated with extensive bilateral consolidations, particularly in the lower

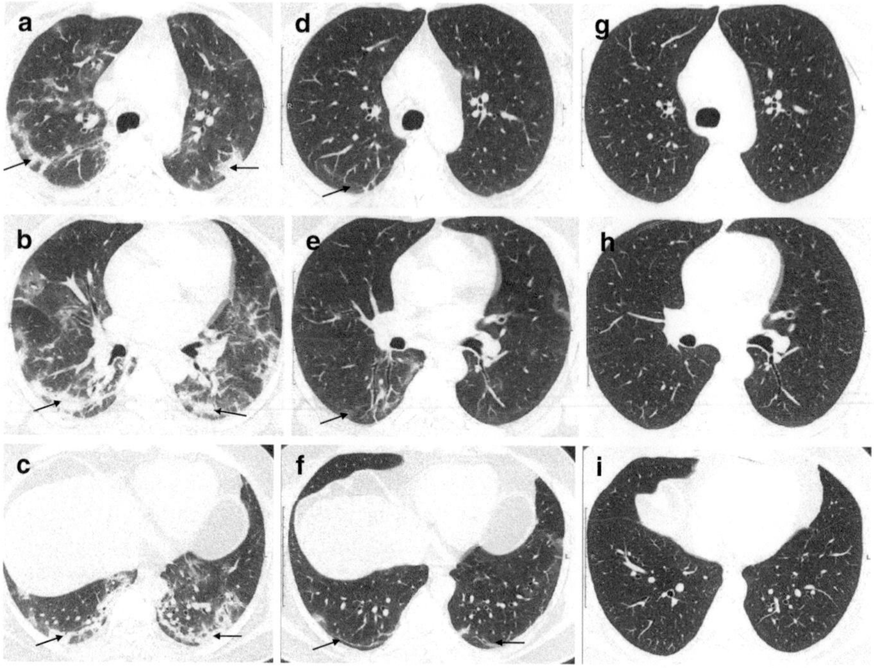

Fig. 3.3 Follow-up CT scans of a 56-year-old male with COVID-19 pneumonia. CT done in the first week of illness shows multifocal subpleural areas of organizing pneumonia (arrows in **a**, **b**, **c**). Follow-up CT done 3 months later (arrows in **d**, **e**, **f**) shows partial resolution with residual subpleural bands, and CT done 1 year later (**g**, **h**, **i**) shows complete resolution

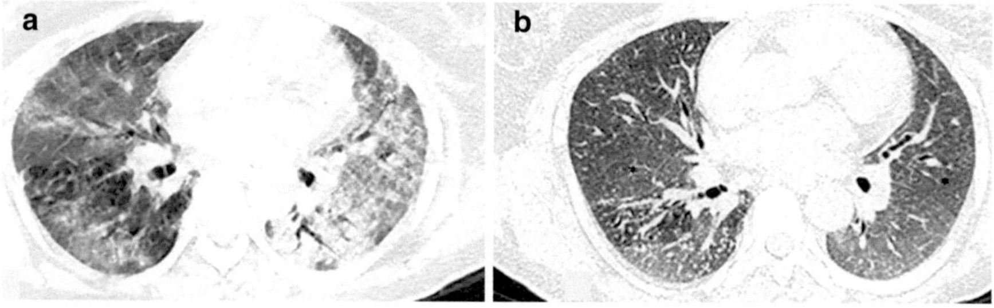

Fig. 3.4 CT features at baseline (**a**) and after 2 months (**b**) in a 45-year-old female who developed severe COVID-19 pneumonia. (**a**) Baseline CT showing bilateral consolidation and ground-glass opacities (GGOs) with peripheral and peribronchovascular distribution. (**b**) Two-month CT follow-up demonstrates resolution of consolidation with a decrease in density but an increase in the extent of GGO marked by * ("tinted sign")

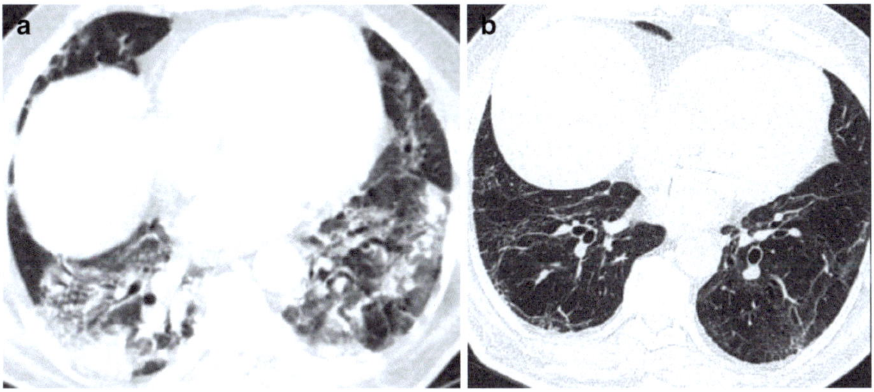

Fig. 3.5 CT features at baseline (**a**) and after 1 year (**b**) in a 73-year-old male who developed severe COVID-19 pneumonia. (**a**) Baseline CT showing bilateral consolidation and ground-glass opacities (GGOs) with peripheral and peribronchovascular distribution. (**b**) One-year CT follow-up demonstrating resolution of consolidation with the appearance of subpleural and parenchymal bands

lobes. In the acute setting or in the few weeks following COVID-19 infection, consolidations can represent bacterial/fungal superinfection as well. Also, a pulmonary infarct resulting from an embolism may manifest as a peripheral area of consolidation.

On follow-up imaging, the sequelae of consolidation will depend on the initial etiology of the consolidation. Acute infective consolidation often resolves faster than areas of GGO. Subparenchymal areas of *linear consolidation* represent the organizing pneumonia phase of inflammation, and as these improve, *parenchymal bands* in similar distribution are seen (Fig. 3.5).

3.2.3 Bronchial Dilatation/Bronchiectasis

Bronchial abnormalities often accompany parenchymal changes in COVID-19 pneumonia. However, it is important to realize that every dilated bronchus should not be labeled as bronchiectasis, as the latter term is reserved for irreversible dilatation. Bronchial dilatation and distortion may be present in areas of GGO or consolidation. It has been shown that as the surrounding parenchymal opacities resolve, this dilatation/distortion may also reverse, although it will be irreversible in some patients wherein fibrosis develops. Hence, it is recommended to use the term *bronchial distortion* instead of "traction bronchiectasis or bronchiolectasis," unless it is established that the changes are irreversible on longer follow-up [6] (Fig. 3.6).

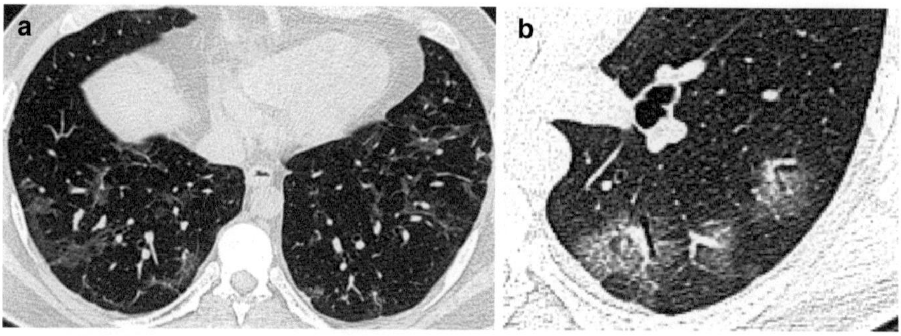

Fig. 3.6 (**a**, **b**) Bronchial dilation/distortion as seen in the areas of GGO in two patients of COVID-19 pneumonia

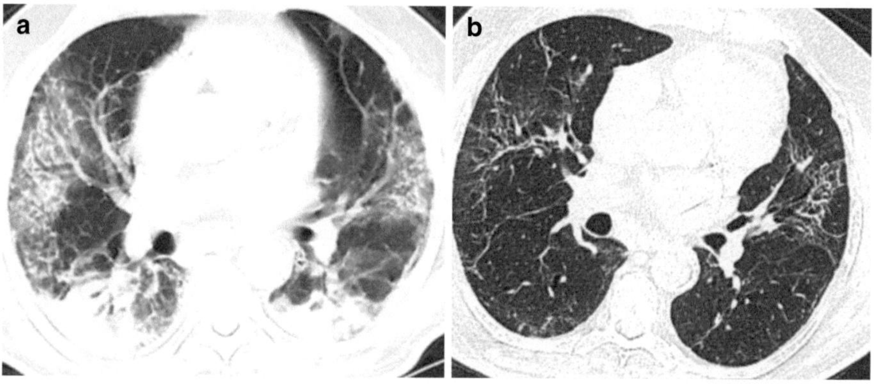

Fig. 3.7 CT features at baseline (**a**) and after 1 year (**b**) in a 73-year-old male who developed severe COVID-19 pneumonia. (**a**) Baseline CT showing bilateral consolidation and ground-glass opacities (GGOs) with peripheral and peribronchovascular distribution. (**b**) One-year CT follow-up demonstrating GGOs and consolidations replaced by areas of fibrotic-like changes showing reticular opacities, interlobular septal thickening with associated bronchial dilation/distortion

3.2.4 Fibrotic-like Changes

In the subacute/late phases of COVID-19 pneumonia, superimposed septal thickening or reticulation may develop on areas of GGO/consolidation with or without associated bronchial dilatation/distortion. Over time, these changes may resolve or evolve into fibrosis. As both potential courses are possible with this appearance, the term *fibrotic-like changes* should be employed at these early time points (initial weeks) rather than fibrosis. No definite timeline has been given for the use of the terminology [6]. These changes can appear relatively early in the course of the disease (as early as the second week) and persist thereafter, particularly in patients with severe disease/ARDS (Fig. 3.7).

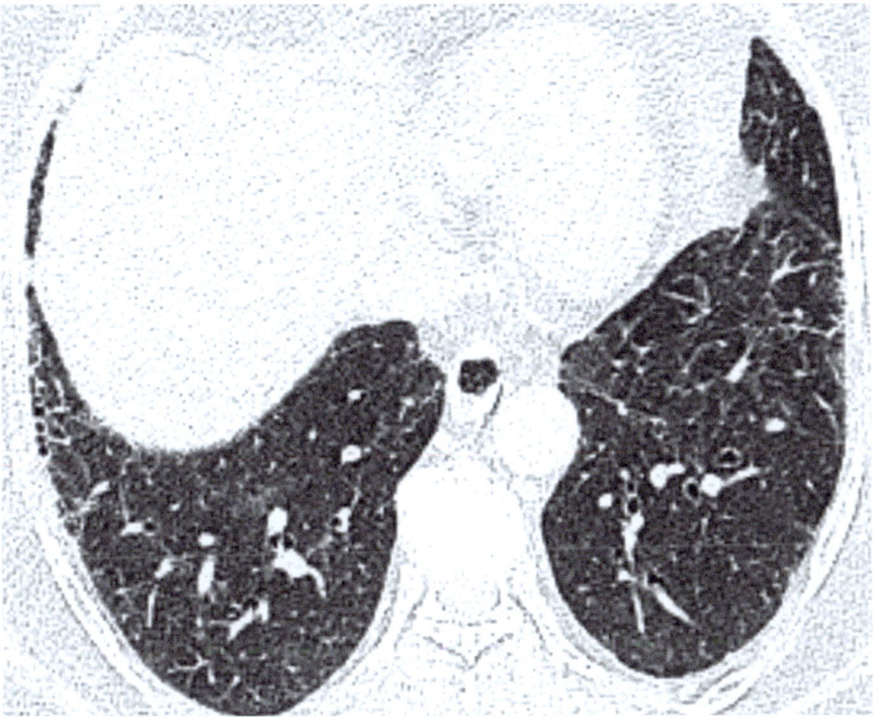

Fig. 3.8 Subpleural areas of fibrosis seen in a follow-up patient of COVID-19 pneumonia in the form of reticular opacities, inter- and intralobular septal thickening, traction bronchiectasis, and subpleural microcysts

3.2.5 Fibrosis

Fibrosis is diagnosed on imaging by the presence of diverse morphology of fibrotic opacities (linear/reticular, parenchymal bands, subpleural lesions) in association with traction bronchiectasis or bronchiolectasis, volume loss, and honey-combing. It has been shown that *fibrotic-like changes of* COVID-19 pneumonia continue to resolve even up to 1 year after the acute event [7, 8]. Hence, the term *fibrosis* can only be employed when the irreversible nature of these lesions has been established. Fibrosis is more likely to develop in those with severe disease/ARDS (Fig. 3.8).

3.2.6 Pulmonary Thromboembolism (PTE) Sequelae

PTE is an established complication of COVID-19. While the thrombus may resolve in most patients, chronic changes may develop in some patients resulting in chronic thromboembolic pulmonary hypertension (CTEPH). These patients will require CT pulmonary angiography (CTPA) studies and echocardiography on follow-up. Besides the large vessels, small-vessel vasculopathy has also been reported in COVID-19 pneumonia; however, its long-term consequence as to whether it could result in pulmonary hypertension is unclear.

3.3 CT Severity Scoring

None of the currently available guidelines recommend a scoring system for radiographs or CT scans performed for patients with post-acute sequelae of COVID-19.

3.4 Various Patterns of Fibrosis/Fibrotic-like Changes

Post-COVID-19 changes may reveal various patterns, some of which are described below:

1. *Subpleural distribution of fibrosis/fibrotic-like changes*: This is the most characteristic pattern observed, as subpleural or peripheral lung zones are the areas that are initially affected most during the acute phase. This pattern subsequently evolves to organizing pneumonia (OP), fibrotic-like changes, and eventually fibrosis. On CT, this morphology resembles nonspecific interstitial pneumonia (NSIP) of interstitial lung disease (ILD). This pattern is particularly confusing in patients with underlying connective tissue diseases (CTDs), as NSIP is the commonest pattern encountered in several CTDs, especially progressive systemic sclerosis and rheumatoid arthritis. In such patients, comparison with previous imaging is the only way of making this distinction [9] (Figs. 3.9 and 3.10).
2. *Peribronchial/central distribution pattern of parenchymal bands*: Although less common than subpleural bands, peribronchial/central distribution of parenchymal bands can also be seen in some patients of post-COVID-19 sequelae (Fig. 3.11).

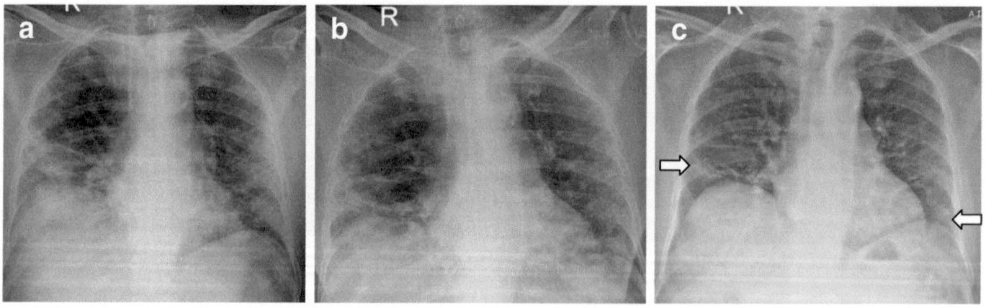

Fig. 3.9 Serial chest radiographs in a 73-year-old male patient with COVID-19 pneumonia. At 1 week of illness (**a**), the CXR shows lower zone and peripheral predominant pneumonia, which shows partial resolution at 6 months (**b**), and at 1 year, (**c**) the chest radiograph shows subpleural fibrotic-like changes (arrows)

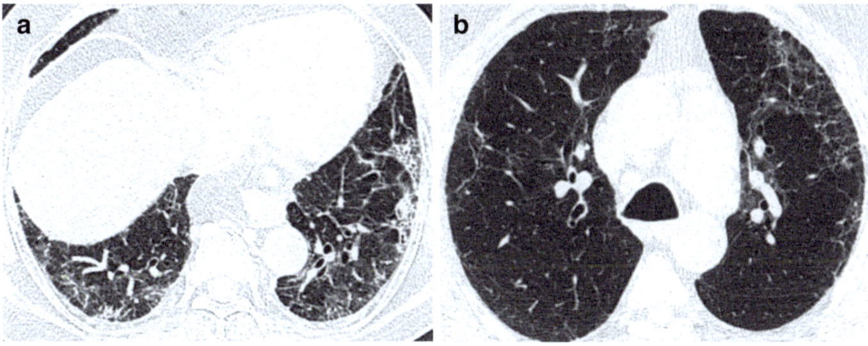

Fig. 3.10 (**a**, **b**) HRCT images of two patients with COVID-19 pneumonia showing predominantly subpleural areas of fibrotic-like changes

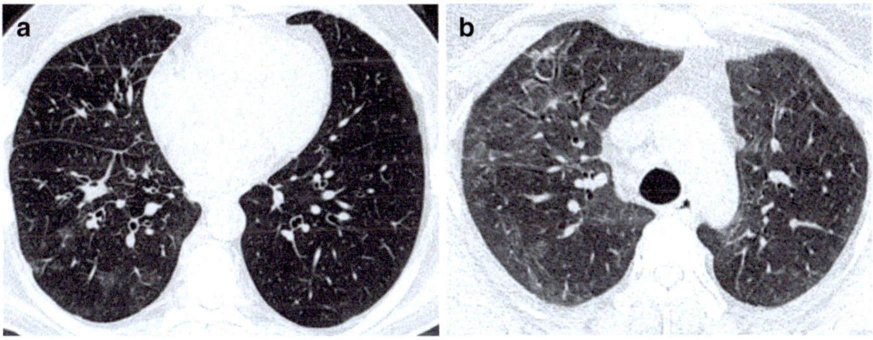

Fig. 3.11 (**a**, **b**) HRCT images of two patients with COVID-19 pneumonia showing predominantly peribronchial areas of fibrotic-like changes along with bronchial wall thickening and bronchial dilation

3. *Fibrosis not conforming to a characteristic distribution*: Often, the distribution of fibrotic-like changes does not conform to a typical subpleural or axial distribution. Parenchymal bands or reticular opacities can be seen in random, asymmetric distribution. In fact, this pattern is primarily post-infective and should not be confused with ILD. It may also be encountered in patients with secondary infections following COVID-19 pneumonia (Fig. 3.12).
4. *Diffuse ground-glass opacities with bronchial dilatation pattern*: While GGOs have been taken as the imaging hallmark of active inflammation in infections or interstitial lung diseases, these can be observed in all phases of pulmonary involvement in COVID-19. This is because GGOs can be the manifestation of pathological changes affecting various compartments of the lung parenchyma, including alveoli, alveolar walls/interstitium, and vascular or airway disorders

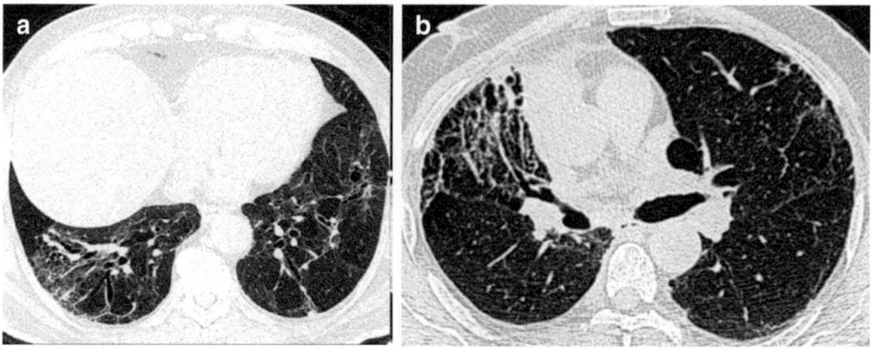

Fig. 3.12 (**a**, **b**) HRCT images of two patients of COVID-19 pneumonia showing both peribronchial and subpleural areas of fibrotic-like changes

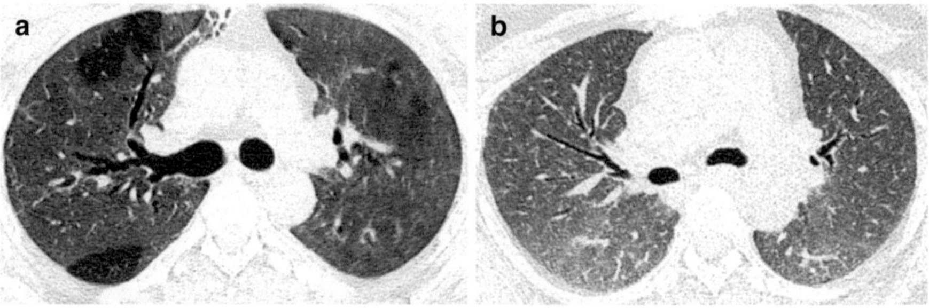

Fig. 3.13 (**a**, **b**) HRCT images of two patients of COVID-19 pneumonia demonstrating diffuse GGOs with associated bronchial dilation

resulting in mosaic attenuation. Lastly, GGO can also result from partial volume artifact of various abnormalities on CT scan. Superadded septal thickening/reticular opacities and dilated bronchi are present when these represent fibrotic-like changes/fibrosis (Fig. 3.13).

5. *Mosaic attenuation*: Mosaic attenuation on CT can be the consequence of either air trapping resulting from constrictive/obliterative bronchiolitis or peripheral vasculopathy. Small airway involvement is seen in several viral pneumonias. Although it is not a signature pattern of COVID-19 pneumonia, it is encountered in several patients. On the other hand, peripheral vasculopathy is well documented in COVID-19 pneumonia resulting in the "vascular tree-in-bud sign" [10]. As long-term sequelae, the mosaic attenuation encountered can be a consequence of both these mechanisms (Fig. 3.14).

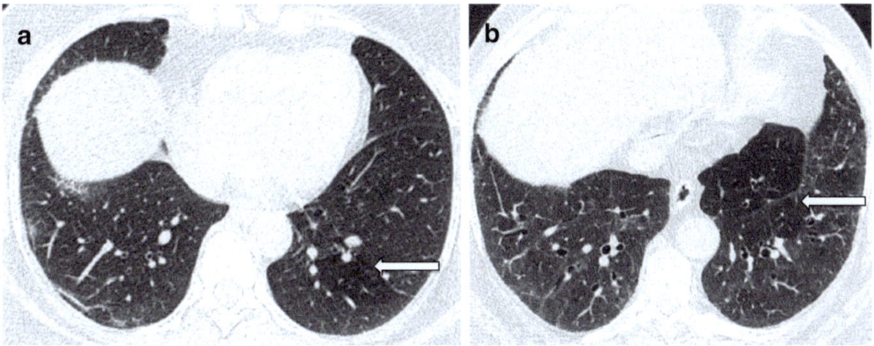

Fig. 3.14 (**a**, **b**) HRCT images of two patients of COVID-19 pneumonia demonstrating areas of low attenuation (arrow) mixed with areas of surrounding high attenuation (mosaic attenuation)

3.5 Conclusion

Based on published literature and institutional experience, it is evident that chest imaging plays an important role in the follow-up of symptomatic patients of post-acute sequelae of COVID-19, as pulmonary fibrosis is a recognized phenotype among these patients. Chest radiographs and spirometry can be used to assess the need for CT scans, and the subsequent frequency of follow-up imaging. CT pulmonary angiography may be required in patients with initial pulmonary thromboembolism during the acute episode. Slow resolution of radiological abnormalities has been documented over up to 1 year following the initial infection and even beyond this period.

References

1. Mylvaganam RJ, Bailey JI, Sznajder JI, Sala MA. Recovering from a pandemic: pulmonary fibrosis after SARS-CoV-2 infection. Eur Respir Rev. 2021;30(162) https://doi.org/10.1183/16000617.0194-2021.
2. Garg M, et al. The conundrum of 'Long-COVID-19': a narrative review. Int J Gen Med. 2021;14:2491–506. https://doi.org/10.2147/ijgm.s316708.
3. BTS Guidance on Respiratory Follow Up of Patients with a Clinico-Radiological Diagnosis of COVID-19 Pneumoniav 1.2 11/5/2020. Accessed.
4. Wang Y, et al. Temporal changes of CT findings in 90 patients with COVID-19 pneumonia: a longitudinal study. Radiology. 2020;296(2):E55–e64. https://doi.org/10.1148/radiol.2020200843.
5. Zhang Z, et al. Temporal lung changes on thin-section CT in patients with COVID-19 pneumonia. Sci Rep. 2020;10(1):19649. https://doi.org/10.1038/s41598-020-76776-x.
6. Martini K, et al. COVID-19 pneumonia imaging follow-up: when and how? A proposition from ESTI and ESR. Eur Radiol. 2021:1–11. https://doi.org/10.1007/s00330-021-08317-7.

7. Han X, et al. Six-month follow-up chest CT findings after severe COVID-19 pneumonia. Radiology. 2021;299(1):E177–e186. https://doi.org/10.1148/radiol.2021203153.
8. Lerum TV, et al. Dyspnoea, lung function and CT findings 3 months after hospital admission for COVID-19. Eur Respir J. 2021;57(4) https://doi.org/10.1183/13993003.03448-2020.
9. Vyas S, Bhalla AS. Imaging conundrum–COVID-related lung changes or connective tissue disease-related interstitial lung disease. Pol J Radiol. 2021;86:e157–8. https://doi.org/10.5114/pjr.2021.104620.
10. Eddy RL, Sin DD. Computed tomography vascular tree-in-bud: a novel prognostic imaging biomarker in COVID-19? Am J Respir Crit Care Med. 2020;202(5):642–4. https://doi.org/10.1164/rccm.202007-2833ED.

Cardiovascular Complications Following COVID-19

4

Ambuj Roy and Aseem Basha M

4.1 Introduction

The ongoing COVID-19 pandemic has affected a huge population of the world, and most of them have made a successful recovery from the acute phase. Survivors of acute illness may experience a wide range of signs and symptoms after recovery which impact their quality of life and add to their disability. These residual sequelae/symptoms are increasingly being reported by recovering patients irrespective of the severity of acute COVID-19 infection. This chapter focusses on cardiovascular complications following COVID-19 infection, common clinical presentations, natural course, evaluation and management in addition to prevention strategies.

4.2 Terminologies Used to Describe Post-acute COVID-19 Phase

In the absence of universally accepted definition, post-COVID-19 syndrome by consensus is defined as signs and symptoms that develop during or after an infection consistent with COVID-19 which continue for more than 12 weeks and are not explained by alternative diagnosis. Common terminologies used are post-COVID-19 syndrome, long-term COVID-19, post-acute sequelae of SARS-CoV-2 (PASC) or long haulers. Also popular in medical fraternity is the term 'long COVID' which is

A. Roy (✉)
Department of Cardiology, All India Institute of Medical Sciences, New Delhi, India

A. Basha M
Department of Cardiology, ABVIMS and Dr. RML Hospital, New Delhi, India

A. Mohan, S. Mittal (eds.), *Post COVID-19 Complications and Management*, https://doi.org/10.1007/978-981-19-4407-9_4

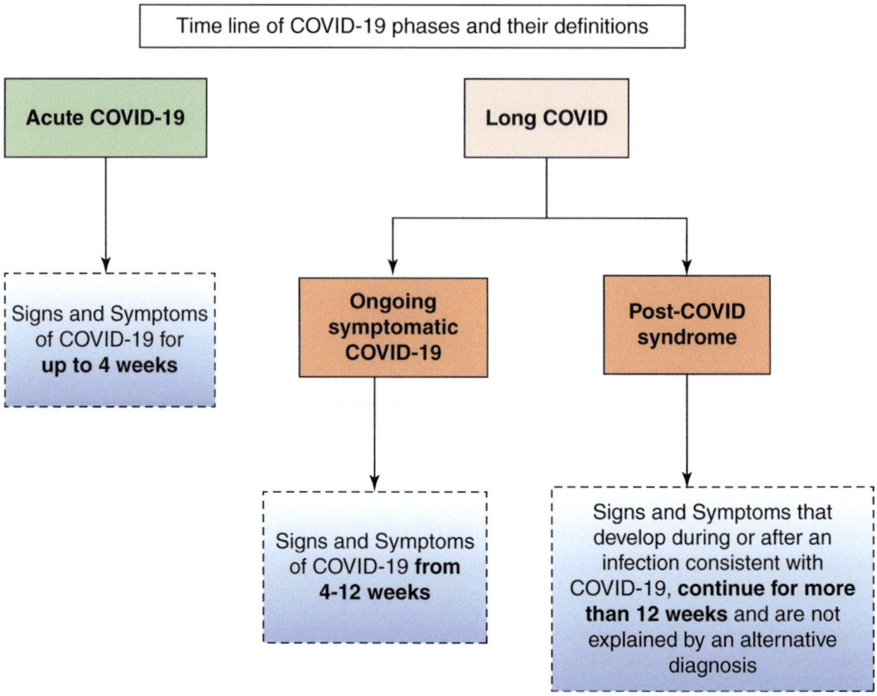

Fig. 4.1 Terminology and definition of acute COVID-19 and long COVID

defined by the National Institute for Health and Care Excellence as symptoms that continue or develop after acute COVID-19. Definitions of various phases of COVID-19 are shown in Figure 4.1 [1–3].

4.3 Cardiovascular Sequelae Post-acute COVID-19 and Pathophysiology

Admitted COVID-19 patients who have survived the acute phase of illness (asymptomatic or symptomatic) seem to have three times greater risk of major adverse cardiovascular events, while mild COVID-19 patients do not seem to have a higher cardiovascular sequelae when matched to controls [4]. However, the focus on cardiovascular sequelae is ever increasing as survivors of acute COVID-19 infection are experiencing persistent symptoms and a decline in quality of life. The risk of cardiovascular sequelae is higher in those requiring hospitalization. This association of increased cardiovascular events post-viral illnesses and post-pandemic has been reported earlier too [5]. Although majority of literature currently is observational with risk of inherent bias, there is considerable evidence pertaining to the symptoms as well as cardiac abnormalities detected on diagnostic testing [6]. While patients with mild or moderate-severe COVID-19 infection are expected to have symptoms of cardiovascular disease lingering on in the post-COVID-19 phase, asymptomatic patients also seem to be variably affected [7]. The spectrum of cardiac manifestations (fatigue, dyspnoea, angina and palpitations) in these long haulers depends not only on the severity of acute COVID-19 infections but also on duration after apparent recovery (Fig. 4.1).

Persistent immune activation post-acute phase, persistent low-grade viremia and residual and ongoing structural/functional changes in myocardium have all been implicated in the pathophysiology of long-term cardiovascular sequelae [8]. A schema of pathophysiology of acute COVID-19 and its subsequent evolution into long-term sequelae is shown in Fig. 4.2. There is considerable heterogeneity in the expression of symptoms and structural/functional abnormalities pertaining to cardiovascular system. Most of the patients having persistent symptoms are usually survivors of mild-moderate acute COVID-19 infection. Few have evidence of cardiac injury evident on cardiac magnetic resonance imaging following mild COVID-19 infection, while those with moderate to severe COVID-19 infection may

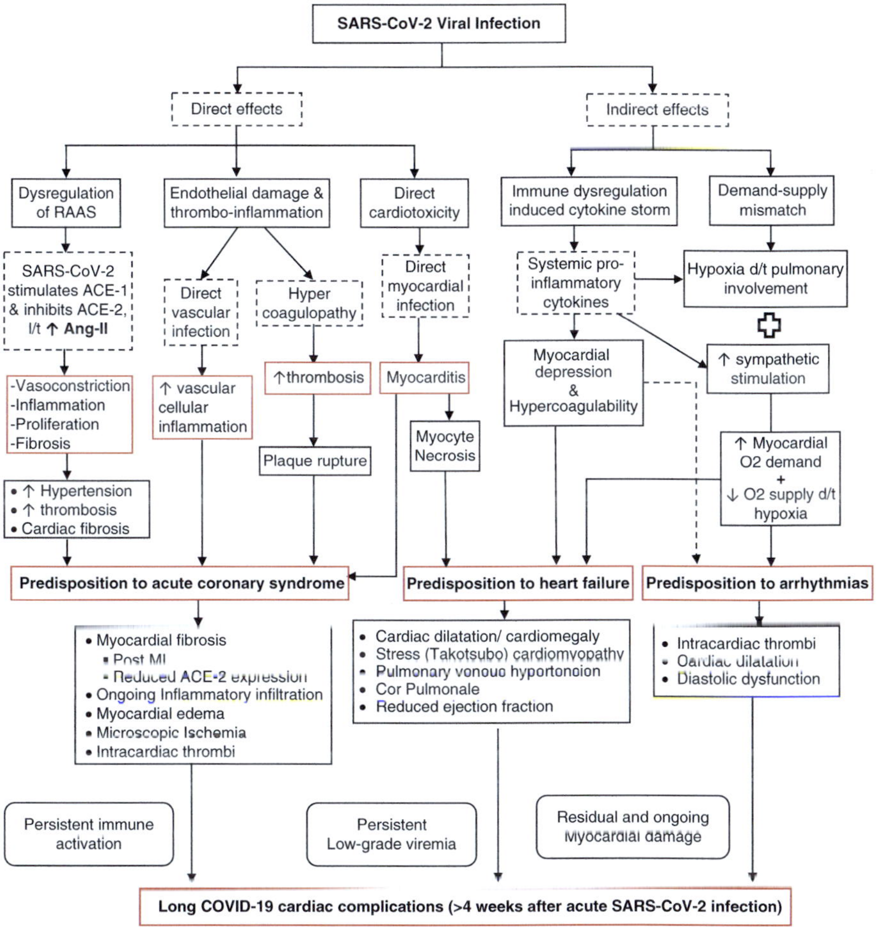

Fig. 4.2 Pathophysiology of long-term cardiovascular sequelae after acute COVID-19 infection

present with biomarker evidence of myocardial injury with or without left ventricular systolic dysfunction. Collateral damage can also be seen in patients presenting late to healthcare facilities with acute cardiac emergencies and culminate into long-lasting/irreversible myocardial injury [9].

4.4 Population at Risk of Post-COVID-19 Sequelae

Patients with severe COVID-19 manifestations, elderly, female sex, poor socioeconomic status, pre-existing comorbidities (diabetes, obesity, coronary artery disease, prior heart failure) and population living in rural areas with poor healthcare services are predisposed to development of long-term cardiac and extracardiac sequelae after apparent recovery [10].

4.5 Cardiovascular Complications Following COVID-19

The long-term sequelae include increased myocardial oxygen demands, irreversible remodelling, myocardial fibrosis/myocardial scar, persistent left ventricular systolic and diastolic dysfunction, heart failure, autonomic dysfunction and arrhythmias. Many of the lingering signs and symptoms seen in patients after they have apparently recovered from acute illness—especially fatigue, dyspnoea, angina and palpitations—appear to have an underlying cardiovascular component. This can occur de novo in an asymptomatic COVID-19 patient or in symptomatic COVID-19 patients with no clinically apparent cardiac involvement during the acute phase. Those who develop viral myocarditis, acute coronary syndrome (ACS), pulmonary embolism (PE), stress-induced cardiomyopathy and arrhythmias during the acute phase are at heightened risk of developing long-term COVID-19 cardiovascular complications and adverse outcomes. These subsets of patients typically have comorbid conditions such as diabetes mellitus, hypertension, obesity, dyslipidaemia and chronic kidney disease which would complicate their recovery after the acute phase.

Up to 20% of patients hospitalized with COVID-19 have clinically significant cardiovascular involvement, while subclinical involvement may be much more common [11, 12]. Epidemiological burden of cardiovascular sequelae post-COVID-19 is variably reported due to inherent bias of observational studies and considerable heterogeneity of studies published. Disproportionate fatigue is the most common symptom in survivors of acute COVID-19. Dyspnoea is by far the second most frequent symptom that persists despite apparent recovery from acute COVID-19 and is multifactorial in aetiology (cardiac, pulmonary or deconditioning to list a few). Prevalence of dyspnoea is reported to be between 22 and 43% in various studies [13].

High index of suspicion of dyspnoea of cardiac origin especially in the setting of ACS, PE, myocarditis and tachyarrhythmias is the key for early diagnosis of worsening cardiac status and initiating appropriate treatment accordingly. Chest pain is reported in survivors of moderate-severe COVID-19 in 18%, 13% [14] and 5% [15] at day 30, day 60 and day 180 of follow-up, respectively. Chest pain consistent with typical angina should be differentiated from atypical or non-anginal chest pain on the basis of quality of pain, aggravating and relieving factors. Palpitations have been noted in 9%, 14% [14] and 9% [16] at day 30, day 60 and day 180 of follow-up, respectively. Differentials for palpitations in post-COVID-19 syndrome include inappropriate sinus tachycardia, postural orthostatic tachycardia syndrome consequent to hyperadrenergic state, or premature ventricular ectopics or ventricular arrhythmias consequent to adverse remodelling, myocardial fibrosis and scarring. Although various tachyarrhythmias and bradyarrhythmias have been reported in acute phase of illness, the prevalence of clinically significant arrhythmias post-recovery from acute illness remains uncertain. Reports of postural orthostatic tachycardia syndrome and autonomic dysfunction have also been reported with COVID-19 as was with other viral illnesses [17]. Although symptoms may be self-limiting for few, most still remain symptomatic beyond 6 months after contracting COVID-19 [16].

A large systematic review of 35 studies published by Ramadan et al [6]. has reported the prevalence of cardiac symptoms and abnormalities (detected on various investigation modalities according to the timeline of evaluation of follow-up) on both short-term and medium-term follow-up. Short-term follow-up (<3 months) has shown prevalence of chest pain, dyspnoea and palpitation to the tune of 25%, 36% and 6%, respectively, while medium-term (3–6 months) follow-up revealed a prevalence of 6%, 3% and 9% for chest pain, dyspnoea and palpitation, respectively (Figs. 4.3 and 4.4). Survivors of acute COVID-19 with cardiovascular

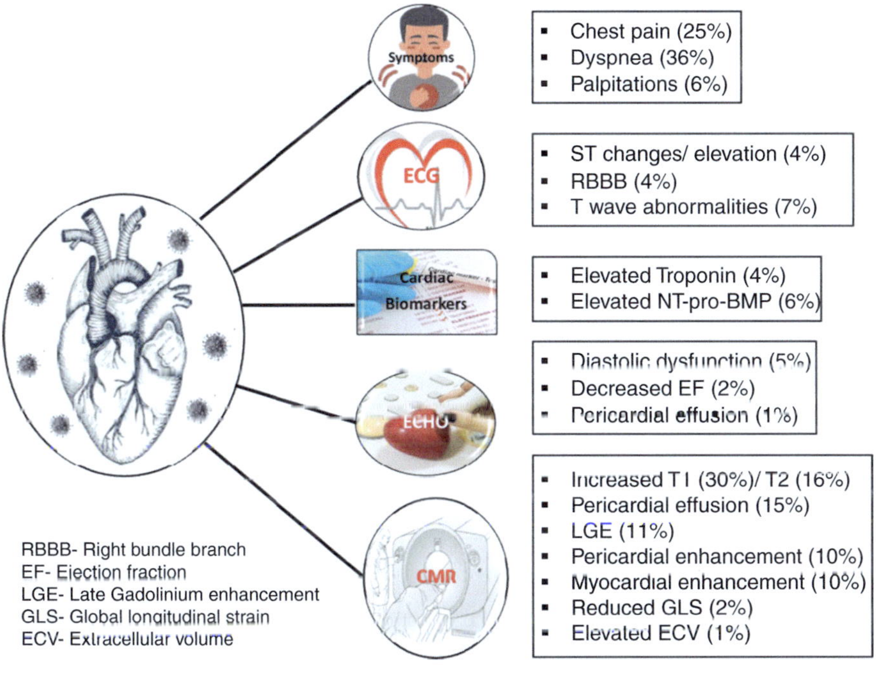

Fig. 4.3 Short-term cardiac sequelae post-COVID-19 (1–3 months) [6]

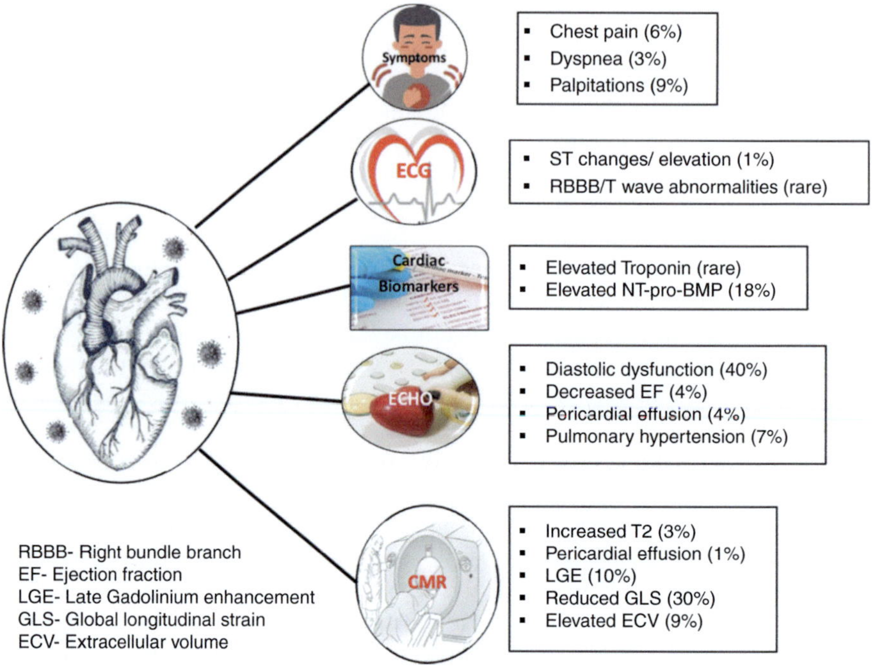

Fig. 4.4 Medium-term cardiac sequelae post-COVID-19 (3–6 months) [6]

events such as myocardial infarction, stroke, venous thromboembolism and arrhythmias would result in symptoms which would persist beyond 6 months (long-term follow-up). However, data is scarce on long-term prevalence of these symptoms.

Two large recently published studies have thrown some light over the long-term sequelae of COVID-19 in the academic year 2022. The first study was 'The Hamburg City Health Study' which followed up patients with mild to moderate SARS-CoV-2 infection for a median period of 9.2 months and looked for cardiac involvement and patient outcomes in comparison to matched cohort. While both echocardiography and cardiac magnetic resonance (CMR)-derived left ventricular systolic function (left ventricular ejection fraction) or right ventricular systolic function (tricuspid annular plane systolic excursion) were numerically reduced in patients with mild to moderate SARS-CoV-2 infection when compared to controls, only the reduction in echocardiography-derived LVEF and TAPSE (tricuspid annular plane systolic excursion) was found to be statistically significant when compared to controls [LVEF, 57.9 vs. 59.1%; regression coefficient −0.93 (95% CI: −1.54,−0.32); adjusted $P = 0.015$; TAPSE, 23.0 vs. 23.9 mm; regression coefficient − 0.72 (95% CI: −1.24, −0.21); adjusted $P = 0.031$, respectively]. Assessment of LVEF and TAPSE by CMR showed no significant differences when compared to controls. Further there were no intergroup differences in other cardiac parameters such as left ventricular diastolic function, peak tricuspid regurgitation velocity and myocardial fibrosis when assessed by CMR [18].

The second study was from the US Department of Veterans Affairs national healthcare database which enrolled a massive cohort of ~1.5 lakh US veterans who survived first 30 days of SARS-CoV-2 infection and were followed up longitudinally for 12 months, and comparison was made with a contemporary cohort and a historical cohort. Estimates of risks and 12-month burden of prespecified incident cardiovascular outcomes in the overall cohort according to nature of care received in the setting of acute infection were calculated. Risks and burdens of individual cardiovascular outcomes are shown in Table 4.1. In this study, the risks and burdens of cardiovascular disease were evident not only in patients who were hospitalized or

Table 4.1 Risks and 12-month burdens of incident post-acute COVID-19 cardiovascular outcomes per 1000 persons compared with the control cohort [19]

Cardiovascular outcome	Risk of outcome (HR (95% CI))	Burden of outcome[a] (HR (95% CI))
Cerebrovascular disorders	1.53 (1.45, 1.61)	5.48 (4.65, 6.35)
• Stroke	1.52 (1.43, 1.62)	4.03 (3.32, 4.79)
• Transient ischemic attacks	1.49 (1.37, 1.62)	1.84 (1.38, 2.34)
Dysrhythmia	1.69 (1.64, 1.75)	19.86 (18.31, 21.46)
• Atrial fibrillation	1.71 (1.64, 1.79)	10.74 (9.61, 11.91)
• Sinus tachycardia	1.84 (1.74, 1.95)	5.78 (5.07, 6.53)
• Sinus bradycardia	1.53 (1.45, 1.62)	4.62 (3.90, 5.38)
• Ventricular arrhythmias	1.84 (1.72, 1.98)	4.18 (3.56, 4.85)
• Atrial flutter	1.80 (1.66, 1.96)	3.10 (2.55, 3.69)
Inflammatory heart disease	2.02 (1.77, 2.30)	1.23 (0.93, 1.57)
• Pericarditis	1.85 (1.61, 2.13)	0.98 (0.70, 1.30)
• Myocarditis	5.38 (3.80, 7.59)	0.31 (0.20, 0.46)
Ischemic heart disease	1.66 (1.52, 1.80)	7.28 (5.80, 8.88)
• Acute coronary disease	1.72 (1.56, 1.90)	5.35 (4.13, 6.70)
• Myocardial infarction	1.63 (1.51, 1.75)	2.91 (2.38, 3.49)
• Ischemic cardiomyopathy	1.75 (1.44, 2.13)	2.34 (1.37, 3.51)
• Angina	1.52 (1.42, 1.64)	2.50 (2.00, 3.03)
Other cardiac disorders	1.72 (1.65, 1.79)	12.72 (11.54, 13.96)
• Heart failure	1.72 (1.65, 1.80)	11.61 (10.47, 12.78)
• Non-ischemic cardiomyopathy	1.62 (1.52, 1.73)	3.56 (2.97, 4.20)
• Cardiac arrest	2.45 (2.08, 2.89)	0.71 (0.53, 0.93)
• Cardiogenic shock	2.43 (1.86, 3.16)	0.51 (0.31, 0.77)
Thrombotic disorders	2.39 (2.27, 2.51)	9.88 (9.05, 10.74)
• Pulmonary embolism	2.93 (2.73, 3.15)	5.47 (4.90, 6.08)
• Deep vein thrombosis	2.09 (1.94, 2.24)	4.18 (3.62, 4.79)
• Superficial vein thrombosis	1.95 (1.80, 2.12)	2.61 (2.20, 3.07)
Major adverse cardiovascular outcome (Composite of myocardial infarction, stroke and all-cause mortality)	1.55 (1.50, 1.60)	23.48 (21.54, 25.48)
Any cardiovascular outcome	1.63 (1.59, 1.68)	45.29 (42.22, 48.45)

[a]Number of excess cases per 1000 individuals

required intensive care but also in those who were not hospitalized. This study highlights the importance of developing an algorithm for early detection of cardiovascular sequelae and institution of timely intervention to mitigate the deleterious effects of this virus on the heart [19].

4.6 Investigations for Evaluation of Cardiovascular Sequelae Post-acute COVID-19

Patients with cardiovascular issues during acute infection or those having signs and symptoms pertaining to cardiac involvement after apparent recovery should be monitored with serial clinical examinations, electrocardiogram, laboratory tests, including cardiac biomarkers (troponin/NT-pro-BNP), and echocardiogram on follow-up visits. Additional diagnostic tests such as cardiac MRI, cardiac pulmonary exercise testing, rhythm monitoring by Holter, chest CT and lower extremity duplex testing are offered according to individual symptoms and examination or test findings, keeping in with clinical standards. Electrocardiogram (ECG), chest radiographs, biomarkers (troponin I, B-type natriuretic peptide), echocardiogram (ECHO) and cardiac magnetic resonance (CMR) imaging have all been used for assessment of cardiac sequelae. Various abnormalities that would suggest cardiovascular involvement on these investigations and their prevalence on short-term and medium-term follow-up have been summarized in Figs. 4.3 and 4.4 [6]. Whether these cardiovascular sequelae detected on various investigations resolve over time or persist forever is yet to be determined and would require long-term follow-up studies. Also, whether patients who have normal troponin levels, ejection fraction and CMR are at increased risk of development of heart failure in future will also require prospective studies to address the same.

4.7 Management

The management of patients with post-COVID-19 cardiac sequelae depends on the status of pre-existing cardiac comorbidities and the cardiac condition developed during the acute phase (ACS, PE, tachy- or bradyarrhythmias, etc.) or during recovery. There is no recommendation currently available for evaluation and management of these patients with varied symptomatology. Hence a careful evaluation with meticulous clinical judgement should guide the modality of investigations in this population. A careful history pertaining to symptoms relevant to cardiovascular sequelae such as dyspnoea, chest pain, palpitation and fatigue should be taken. It should be determined whether symptoms are of new onset, persistent or worsening of pre-existing symptoms. Clinical examination in these patients should focus on vital signs (heart rate, blood pressure and saturation), and patient should also be checked for postural hypotension in patients presenting with presyncope or syncope. A systematic cardiovascular system examination for murmurs, pericardial rub, abnormal diastolic heart sounds, jugular venous pressure and signs of pulmonary oedema should be looked for.

Patients with new-onset or persistent dyspnoea or worsening of pre-existing dyspnoea should undergo chest radiograph to differentiate cardiac versus pulmonary causes of dyspnoea. Cardiopulmonary exercise testing (CPX) can further help in differentiating the aetiology of dyspnoea (cardiac versus pulmonary versus deconditioning). Patients with fatigue and palpitations should have a baseline 12-lead ECG with Holter reserved only for patients having an unremarkable baseline ECG. Echocardiogram should not be routinely performed and is reserved for those patients with history or biomarker evidence of myocardial injury, orthopnea, abnormal jugular venous or auscultatory findings or abnormal chest X-ray or ECG. Although CMR can be used to detect myocarditis that was not evident in acute phase, its clinical utility is questionable, and routine use of CMR for detecting myocardial injury should be strongly discouraged.

Symptom-guided investigations and appropriate guideline directed medical therapy (GDMT) in patients with predisposing or perpetuating factors such as diabetes mellitus, hypertension, obesity, atrial fibrillation and prior ACS and heart failure are key for optimal outcomes in these patients. Patients (nonathletes) with symptoms but no abnormalities on imaging should be advised on dos and don'ts during the post-COVID-19 phase. The dos include restructuring of daily routines, emphasis on maintaining healthy weight, moderate-intensity exercise (30 min per day, five times a week), meditation/yoga, vaccination 3 months post-recovery (if not previously vaccinated) and avoidance of alcohol/smoking/self-medications. Patients with persistent symptoms (such as fatigue, cough, breathlessness, fever) should limit activity to 60% of maximum heart rate until 2–3 weeks after symptoms resolve, while they should refrain from intense cardiovascular exercise for up to 3 months after myocarditis or pericarditis [20].

Anecdotal reports of sudden cardiac deaths after resumption of their active lifestyle post-recovery have stirred an active debate regarding whether routine echocardiograms/CMR/coronary angiograms should be performed prior to resumption of active lifestyle. Routine investigation of these apparently healthy adults is neither recommended nor warranted. Athletes post-COVID-19 who have evidence of exercise-induced cardiac remodelling (physiological) with no ongoing clinical concerns and normal ECG and biomarkers should be permitted for graded return to play. In those with ongoing clinical concerns, CMR and other secondary imaging modalities as directed by clinical suspicion should be performed and pathologies appropriately treated before resumption of athletic activities [21]. An algorithm for evaluating patients with cardiac sequelae and their management is shown in Fig. 4.5.

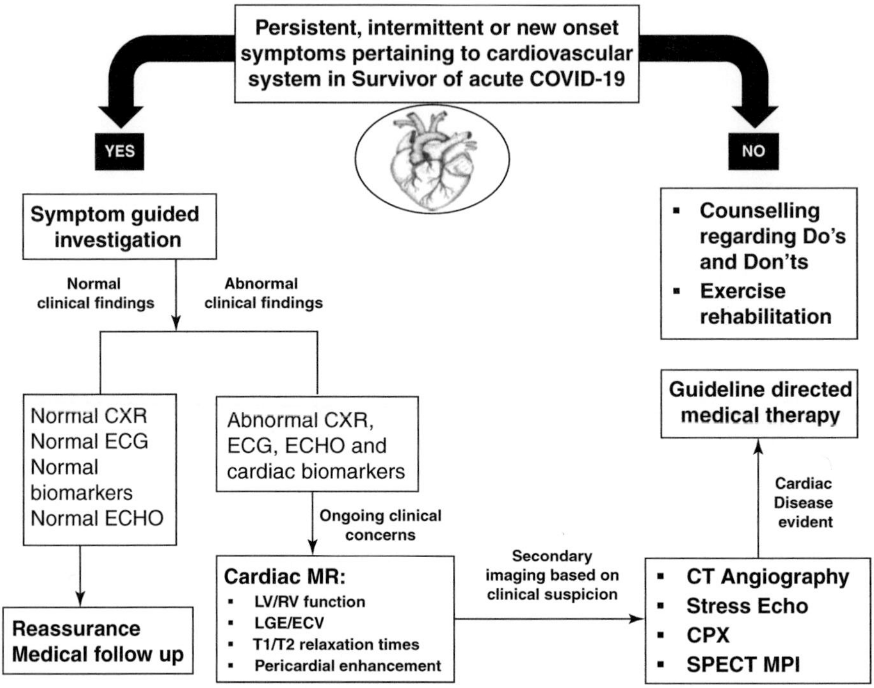

Fig. 4.5 Algorithm for evaluation and management of post-COVID-19 sequelae

4.8 Prevention Strategies

The most cost-effective strategy would be vaccination to prevent from acute COVID-19 in the first place in addition to hand hygiene and social distancing. Also, in survivors of acute infection with persistent or ongoing symptoms, vaccination (after COVID-19) has been reported with resolution of these symptoms [22]. Telephonic follow-up in patients with persistent symptoms and outpatient follow-up visits for those with underlying predisposing factors will help in early diagnosis and treatment of these long haulers. All patients post-discharge should be monitored for cardiovascular risk factors like tobacco use, high blood pressure, raised blood sugars and dyslipidaemia. Diligent management of these risk factors is mandatory to reduce the heightened risk of major adverse cardiovascular events in them. All patients with pre-existing atherosclerotic cardiovascular disease should also be on aspirin and statins as per standard guidelines.

4.9 Conclusion

On completion of 2 years of the pandemic, we are now experiencing an ever-increasing population who have survived the pandemic but have persistent, intermittent or new-onset symptoms pertaining to cardiovascular system. Pathophysiology of these cardiac sequelae is complex and multifactorial. Careful identification of predisposing factors, meticulous history, examination and clinically directed investigations help us in early diagnosis and treatment of these patients.

4.10 Take-Home Message

- Cardiovascular sequelae are seen in patients with previous cardiac comorbidities and also seen in healthy survivors of acute illness including those with mild COVID-19.
- Admitted patients of COVID-19 have three times higher probability of major adverse cardiovascular events including heart failure, acute coronary syndrome and cardiovascular mortality.
- Diligent management of cardiovascular risks like blood pressure, diabetes, dyslipidaemia and lifestyle is needed in survivors of COVID-19 to reduce major adverse cardiovascular events.
- Cardiac investigations in these predisposed populations should be clinically driven.
- Exercise prescription post-acute COVID-19 should be individualized to prevent worsening of cardiac symptoms and sudden cardiac deaths.

References

1. Greenhalgh T, Knight M, A'Court C, Buxton M, Husain L. Management of post-acute covid-19 in primary care. BMJ. 2020 Aug 11;370:m3026.
2. Shah W, Hillman T, Playford ED, Hishmeh L. Managing the long term effects of covid-19: summary of NICE, SIGN, and RCGP rapid guideline. BMJ. 2021 Jan 22;372:n136.
3. Venkatesan P. NICE guideline on long COVID. Lancet Respir Med. 2021 Feb 1;9(2):129.
4. Joy G, Artico J, Kurdi H, et al. Prospective case-control study of cardiovascular abnormalities 6 months following mild COVID-19 in healthcare workers. JACC Cardiovasc Imaging. 2021;14(11):2155–66. https://doi.org/10.1016/j.jcmg.2021.04.011.
5. Public Health Weekly Reports for November 11, 1932. Public Health Rep. 1932 Nov 11;47(46):2159–89.
6. Ramadan MS, Bertolino L, Zampino R, Durante-Mangoni E. Cardiac sequelae after coronavirus disease 2019 recovery: a systematic review. Clin Microbiol Infect. 2021 Sep;27(9):1250–61.

7. Augustin M, Schommers P, Stecher M, Dewald F, Gieselmann L, Gruell H, et al. Post-COVID syndrome in non-hospitalised patients with COVID-19: a longitudinal prospective cohort study. Lancet Reg Health Eur. 2021 Jul;6:100122.
8. Ramakrishnan RK, Kashour T, Hamid Q, Halwani R, Tleyjeh IM. Unraveling the mystery surrounding post-acute sequelae of COVID-19. Front Immunol. 2021 Jun 30;12:686029.
9. Satterfield BA, Bhatt DL, Gersh BJ. Cardiac involvement in the long-term implications of COVID-19. Nat Rev Cardiol. 2021 Oct 22:1–10.
10. Jiang DH, Roy DJ, Gu BJ, Hassett LC, McCoy RG. Postacute sequelae of severe acute respiratory syndrome coronavirus 2 infection: a state-of-the-art review. JACC Basic Transl Sci. 2021 Oct;6(9):796–811.
11. Yancy CW, Fonarow GC. Coronavirus disease 2019 (COVID-19) and the heart-is heart failure the next chapter? JAMA Cardiol. 2020 Nov 1;5(11):1216–7.
12. Puntmann VO, Carerj ML, Wieters I, Fahim M, Arendt C, Hoffmann J, et al. Outcomes of cardiovascular magnetic resonance imaging in patients recently recovered from coronavirus disease 2019 (COVID-19). JAMA Cardiol. 2020 Nov 1;5(11):1265–73.
13. Nalbandian A, Sehgal K, Gupta A, Madhavan MV, McGroder C, Stevens JS, et al. Post-acute COVID-19 syndrome. Nat Med. 2021 Apr;27(4):601–15.
14. Carvalho-Schneider C, Laurent E, Lemaignen A, Beaufils E, Bourbao-Tournois C, Laribi S, et al. Follow-up of adults with noncritical COVID-19 two months after symptom onset. Clin Microbiol Infect Off Publ Eur Soc Clin Microbiol Infect Dis. 2021 Feb;27(2):258–63.
15. Carfì A, Bernabei R, Landi F. Gemelli against COVID-19 post-acute care study group. Persistent symptoms in patients after acute COVID-19. JAMA. 2020 Aug 11;324(6):603–5.
16. Huang C, Huang L, Wang Y, Li X, Ren L, Gu X, et al. 6-month consequences of COVID-19 in patients discharged from hospital: a cohort study. Lancet Lond Engl. 2021 Jan 16;397(10270):220–32.
17. Blitshteyn S, Whitelaw S. Postural orthostatic tachycardia syndrome (POTS) and other autonomic disorders after COVID-19 infection: a case series of 20 patients. Immunol Res. 2021 Apr;69(2):205–11.
18. Petersen EL, Goßling A, Adam G, Aepfelbacher M, Behrendt C-A, Cavus E, et al. Multi-organ assessment in mainly non-hospitalized individuals after SARS-CoV-2 infection: the Hamburg City health study COVID programme. Eur Heart J. 2022 Jan 6:ehab914.
19. Xie Y, Xu E, Bowe B, Al-Aly Z. Long-term cardiovascular outcomes of COVID-19. Nat Med 2022 Feb 7;
20. Barker-Davies RM, O'Sullivan O, Senaratne KPP, Baker P, Cranley M, Dharm-Datta S, et al. The Stanford hall consensus statement for post-COVID-19 rehabilitation. Br J Sports Med. 2020 Aug;54(16):949–59.
21. Phelan D, Kim JH, Elliott MD, Wasfy MM, Cremer P, Johri AM, et al. Screening of potential cardiac involvement in competitive athletes recovering from COVID-19: an expert consensus statement. JACC Cardiovasc Imaging. 2020 Dec;13(12):2635–52.
22. Arnold DT, Milne A, Samms E, Stadon L, Maskell NA, Hamilton FW. Are vaccines safe in patients with Long COVID? A prospective observational study. Preprint. posted online March 14, 2021. medRxiv. 2021. https://doi.org/10.1101/2021.03.11.21253225.

Neurological Sequelae of COVID-19 5

M. V. Padma Srivastava and Ayush Agarwal

Learning Points

1. Neurological complications/sequelae of COVID-19 may occur both in the para-infectious and post-infectious phase and may be independent of respiratory manifestations.
2. Stroke, headache, and immune-mediated phenomenon are the most common post-COVID-19 neurological manifestations.
3. Early diagnosis and treatment are essential for a good functional outcome.

5.1 Introduction

SARS-CoV-2 belongs to the family of coronaviruses known to cause respiratory, gastrointestinal, and enteric infections. They are single-stranded enveloped viruses and derive their name from the Latin word *corona*, meaning crown (resemblance due to the spike proteins on the viral surface). These viruses can be classified into four genera: *Alphacoronavirus*, *Betacoronavirus*, *Deltacoronavirus*, and *Gammacoronavirus*, of which the first three infect mammals. Human infection is usually mild; occasionally, however, the virus jumps between species leading to the emergence of lethal strains like Middle East respiratory syndrome (MERS) coronavirus and severe acute respiratory syndrome (SARS) coronavirus (SARS-CoV-1 and SARS-CoV-2) [1].

SARS-CoV-2 has four major structural proteins: spike, membrane, envelope, and nucleocapsid. The spike protein is used for attachment to various receptors in the human body like ACE2 and neuropilin [2]. COVID-19 is the clinical disease caused by SARS-CoV-2 infection and was first reported in December 2019 in Wuhan,

M. V. P. Srivastava (✉) · A. Agarwal
Department of Neurology, All India Institute of Medical Sciences, New Delhi, India

A. Mohan, S. Mittal (eds.), *Post COVID-19 Complications and Management*,
https://doi.org/10.1007/978-981-19-4407-9_5

China. However, within months it spread across the globe, posing the biggest challenge to humanity in this century leading to more than 600 million infections and 6 million deaths worldwide as on mid-September 2022 [3].

5.2 Neurological Sequelae of COVID-19

Approximately 10–35% of survivors of COVID-19 develop persistent disabling neurological sequelae [4]. Considering the enormity of the number of infections, the burden of long-term neurological complications is unfathomable. Thus, it is essential to be acutely aware of these conditions for early diagnosis and management to prevent irreversible long-term sequelae.

The neurological manifestations of COVID-19 can broadly be divided into para-infectious complications (those occurring during the acute infection phase) and post-acute phase complications. A list of the common manifestations is depicted in Table 5.1.

5.2.1 Anosmia and Ageusia

These are often the heralding manifestations of infection. Anosmia occurs in approximately 40–60% of cases, but some alteration in smell (upon testing) is present in 90% of infected individuals [5, 6]. Ageusia is secondary to the loss of smell and often leads to loss of appetite and weight. These symptoms are usually transient and recover within 1–8 weeks. This is because the disruption of the olfactory nerve does not occur and the symptoms result from an infection of the sustentacular cells leading to temporary olfactory cleft obstruction and edema of the olfactory bulb [4]. However, some individuals develop persistent hyposmia, anosmia or hypo-/ageusia.

Table 5.1 Neurological complications of COVID-19

Para-infectious	• Anosmia and ageusia • Encephalopathy • Stroke • Encephalitis • Myositis • Seizures • Headache
Post-infectious	• ADEM • GBS • Myelitis • Seizures • Long-haul COVID • Multisystem inflammatory syndrome

5.2.2 Encephalopathy

This is the commonest neurological manifestation in hospitalized patients with COVID-19. Approximately 30–35% of patients develop encephalopathic manifestations (commoner with old age) ranging from seizures to delirium and altered mental status [4]. The cause for these manifestations is manifold and includes hypoxia, multi-organ involvement, metabolic abnormalities, direct central nervous system (CNS) involvement, drugs like corticosteroids and sedatives, and finally, separation from family members. These individuals often have prolonged hospital stay, and the majority is not independent for activities of daily living upon discharge [7]. Magnetic resonance imaging (MRI) of the brain may reveal micro-hemorrhagic lesions involving the corpus callosum and juxtacortical regions or diffuse, bilateral hyperintense lesions involving the ganglio-capsular region (post-hypoxia) [8]. Encephalopathy due to reversible causes like drugs, sepsis, or metabolic abnormalities recovers with supportive treatment.

Acute necrotizing hemorrhagic encephalopathy is a severe and often lethal variant that is believed to occur secondary to cytokine release syndrome (cytokine storm) and not direct infection by SARS-CoV-2. The cytokine storm disrupts the blood-brain barrier and causes necrosis of the brain. Afflicted individuals present with rapidly progressive altered sensorium, and MRI brain typically reveals bilateral hemorrhagic lesions involving the thalami, temporal lobes, and brainstem. Treatment response to intravenous immunoglobulin (IVIg) and plasma exchange is usually poor.

5.2.3 Viral Encephalitis

This is an uncommon manifestation of COVID-19 infection as direct invasion of the brain has been rarely described. Even in suspected cases, cerebrospinal fluid (CSF) or autopsy studies on brain parenchyma failed to demonstrate the presence of SARS-CoV-2 RNA and proteins [9, 10]. The severity of neuropathological changes was also not associated with presence of the virus.

5.2.4 Acute Disseminated Encephalomyelitis (ADEM)

ADEM is known to occur post-viral infections and is commoner in children. However, post-COVID-19 ADEM has predominantly been described in adults following a mild flu-like presentation and severe COVID-19 warranting intensive care [11]. Patients usually present with multifocal deficits and encephalopathy, and MRI brain reveals T2/FLAIR asymmetrical hyperintensities involving the white matter (deep and gray-white interface) [4]. Occasionally, hemorrhagic changes can occur concomitantly. SARS-CoV-2 is undetectable in the CSF of these patients, and management with high-dose corticosteroids leads to good treatment response. Hemorrhagic ADEM complicates management of COVID-19 by preventing anticoagulant treatment or thromboprophylaxis, which is usually otherwise warranted in these patients.

5.2.5 Stroke

The Virchow's triad is a combination of hypercoagulable state, endothelial dysfunction, and immobility [4]. SARS-CoV-2 causes cerebrovascular complications through all three mechanisms, and strokes have been reported in 5% of COVID-19 patients. Older patients with concomitant atherosclerotic risk factors are at higher risk. Ischemic (most common) [Fig. 5.1] and hemorrhagic strokes, as well as cerebral venous sinus thrombosis, are now known to occur with and due to SARS-CoV-2 [12]. Hypercoagulable state results from impaired fibrinolysis, antiphospholipid antibodies, high levels of coagulation factors, and low level of anticoagulants. This can be demonstrated by elevations of D-dimer levels, prothrombin time, and activated partial thromboplastin times [13], and such patients are treated with prophylactic anticoagulants to prevent these events. Endothelial injury mediated by SARS-CoV-2 results in depletion of nitric oxide synthase leading to subsequent deficiency of nitric oxide (potent vasodilator and inhibitor of leucocyte and platelet adhesion to the endothelium) [14]. ACE2 binding of SARS-CoV-2

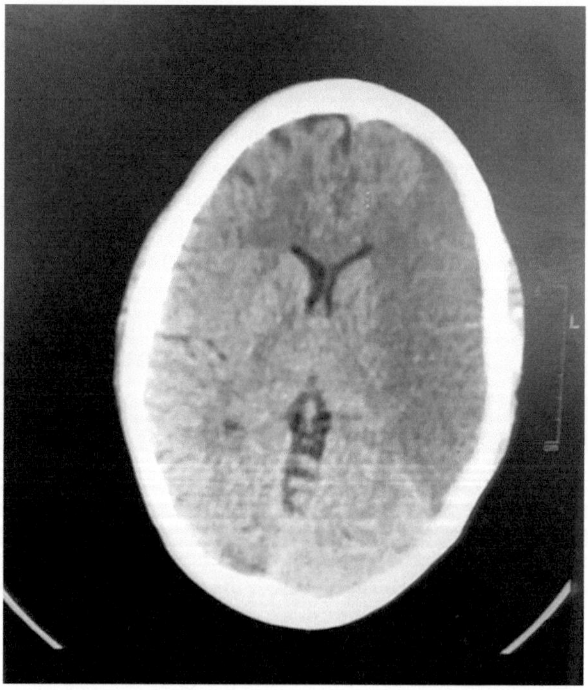

Fig. 5.1 Non-contrast CT head of a SARS-CoV-2-infected patient with a malignant left middle cerebral artery infarct

also leads to reduced expression of the former, leading to unregulated angiotensin II levels (a potent vasoconstrictor), eventually causing increased hypertension and, therefore, stroke risk. COVID-19-associated inflammatory response also predisposes to plaque rupture in patients with the pre-existing atherosclerotic disease [14].

All acute ischemic strokes (eligible for thrombolysis) are treated in the same manner as non-COVID-19-associated events. However, some clinicians prefer tenecteplase over alteplase in this setting because of the former's more rapid onset of effect and bolus dosage.

5.2.6 Neurodegenerative Diseases

COVID-19-associated cases of acute parkinsonism and one case of Creutzfeldt-Jakob disease have been reported till date [15, 16]. However, it is unclear and debatable whether SARS-CoV-2 infection was causative or coincidental or whether the inflammatory response elicited due to its infection precipitated these neurodegenerative diseases. There is no evidence of acceleration of these diseases or increased susceptibility to them after SARS-CoV-2 infection. However, whether these eventually occur as a long-term sequela remains to be seen since ACE2 expression within the CNS is high.

5.2.7 Myelitis

Multiple cases of acute myelitis following SARS-CoV-2 infection have been described, with acute transverse myelitis involving three or more contiguous segments being the commonest form. MRI spine shows longitudinally extensive gray and white matter involvement, although normal MRIs (MRI-negative myelitis) can also be encountered [17]. These patients usually respond to treatment with plasma exchange and steroids. Occasionally, a more severe acute necrotizing myelitis has also been reported.

5.2.8 Guillain-Barré Syndrome (GBS)

Multiple cases of post-COVID-19 GBS have been described, with the onset of GBS symptoms occurring 5–10 days after the development of COVID-19 symptoms [18]. It results from molecular mimicry between antigens of SARS-CoV-2 and antigens of the peripheral nerve. However, the virus could not be detected in the CSF of any patient, and both demyelinating and axonal variants have been reported. In addition, there was a slight increase in the proportion of patients presenting with rarer variants such as the Miller Fisher variant. Most cases had albumin-cytological dissociation and responded well to IVIg and plasma exchange treatment. The former was preferred due to ease of administration and noninvasiveness, especially in the background of COVID-19.

5.2.9 Myositis

The development of myositis is associated with muscle weakness and myalgia that can occur at any point during the course of the illness and can persist after recovery of all other symptoms [19]. Limb muscle involvement is most common, but paraspinal involvement is also reported and can lead to back or abdominal pain. Severe affliction may lead to rhabdomyolysis. MRI of the affected muscles shows swelling and occasionally may reveal features suggestive of myonecrosis. Patients usually respond well to intravenous corticosteroids.

5.2.10 Long-haul COVID with Neurological Manifestations

This syndrome is independent of the severity of the acute manifestations and can even occur in patients with minimal/mild symptoms [20]. It is commoner in milder disease, and one hypothesis states that since these patients did not get admitted, they might not have adequately cleared the virus leading to restricted or persistent viral replication leading to this syndrome. The symptomatology overlaps with chronic fatigue syndrome and is more common in young adults and women. Three common subtypes include the following:

- *Predominant dysautonomia*—Patients present with palpitations, hypo- or hypertension, tachycardia on mild exertion, gastroparesis, diarrhea, or constipation.
- *Extreme exercise intolerance*—Patients complain of extreme tiredness and fatigue, significantly limiting physical activity out of proportion to the previous state of health.
- *Cognitive impairment*—Patients present with sleep disturbance (31%), short-term memory dysfunction (34%), distortion of time and place, or depression.

The exact extent of this syndrome is unknown. A distinction between long-haul COVID with lingering symptoms due to severe COVID-19-associated multi-organ dysfunction should always be made prior to diagnosis with the former.

5.2.11 Multisystem Inflammatory Syndrome (in Children)

Some children develop systemic symptoms 2–3 weeks after recovery from acute COVID-19 illness, including neurological symptoms [4]. The exact pathophysiology is unclear, and common symptoms include generalized weakness, dysarthria/dysphagia, and encephalopathy. Blood investigations reveal elevated inflammatory markers, but CSF is normal. MRI brain may sometimes reveal diffusion restriction involving the splenium of the corpus callosum. Patients usually have a good response to IVIg and steroids.

5.2.12 Headache

This is one of the commonest CNS manifestations and occurs in 6–25% of patients with COVID-19 [14]. The headache is usually moderate-severe in intensity and occurs due to the systemic spread of the virus and its associated inflammation. Other causes include anxiety, isolation, and decreased sleep. Most patients with headaches have a previous history of headaches as well. However, some cases develop new-onset headache peri- or post-COVID-19 infection. The headache usually responds well to analgesics.

5.2.13 Seizures

SARS-CoV-2 infection decreases the seizure threshold leading to worsening seizure control/frequency in epileptic patients or causing seizures in individuals with no prior history. Mechanisms by which seizures can occur include COVID-19-associated brain damage, encephalitis or meningoencephalitis, and pro-inflammatory milieu [14]. Seizures can even be the first presenting symptom of SARS-CoV-2 infection and may be either focal or generalized. Management of seizures is the same as that of COVID-19-negative patients. However, drug-drug interactions must be considered since many anti-epileptic drugs induce or inhibit cytochrome CYP systems leading to altered pharmacogenetics of COVID-19 drugs (CYP inducers like phenytoin and carbamazepine will decrease the plasma concentration, whereas CYP inhibitors like valproate will increase the plasma concentration of drugs used for the treatment of COVID-19).

5.2.14 Dizziness

Dizziness occurs in approximately 8–9% of subjects post-COVID-19, and the exact pathophysiology in this setting is poorly understood. Some retrospective observational studies have described it as one of the most common neurologic findings in SARS-CoV-2 infection, and therefore clinicians should be vigilant about this symptom, even in the absence of prototypical respiratory symptoms.

5.2.15 Neurological Complications of Vaccination

Most vaccines against COVID-19 are based on the virus spike protein delivered as DNA, mRNA, or protein. Although they have demonstrated excellent safety and efficacy profiles, neurological complications may rarely occur following vaccination. Multiple cases of Bell's palsy and a few cases of myelitis, ADEM, stroke, and GBS have been reported following vaccination with different vaccines worldwide, although definite causality has not been proven. Vaccine-associated thrombotic thrombocytopenia has also been reported with associated antibodies against platelet factor 4 (similar to heparin-induced thrombotic thrombocytopenia), and these patients should not be treated with IVIg and non-heparin-based anticoagulants.

5.3 Conclusion

Neurological complications from SARS-CoV-2 can occur both during and post-acute phases of the disease. Clinical awareness and knowledge of these conditions are essential since early recognition and treatment usually lead to good outcomes. The occurrence of long-term sequelae in the form of neurodegenerative diseases will only be known through long-term follow-up of these patients.

Conflict of Interest None

Financial Disclosures None

References

1. Li Y, Li H, Fan R, et al. Coronavirus infections in the central nervous system and respiratory tract show distinct features in hospitalized children. Intervirology. 2016;59(3):163–9. https://doi.org/10.1159/000453066.
2. Lu Y, Gong EC, Zhang QY, et al. Expression of SARS-CoV in various types of cells in lung tissues [in Chinese]. Beijing Da XueXue Bao Yi Xue Ban. 2005;37(5):453–7.
3. www.covid19.who.int
4. Nath A. Neurologic manifestations of severe acute respiratory syndrome coronavirus 2 infection. Continuum. 2021;27(4, Neuroinfectious Disease):1051–65.
5. Lechien JR, Chiesa-Estomba CM, De Siati DR, et al. Olfactory and gustatory dysfunctions as a clinical presentation of mild-to-moderate forms of the coronavirus disease (COVID-19): a multicenter European study. Eur Arch Otorhinolaryngol. 2020;277(8):2251–61. https://doi.org/10.1007/s00405-020-05965-1.
6. Hornuss D, Lange B, Schröter N, et al. Anosmia in COVID-19 patients. Clin Microbiol Infect. 2020;26(10):1426–7. https://doi.org/10.1016/j.cmi.2020.05.017.
7. Liotta EM, Batra A, Clark JR, et al. Frequent neurologic manifestations and encephalopathy-associated morbidity in Covid-19 patients. Ann Clin Transl Neurol. 2020;7(11):2221–30. https://doi.org/10.1002/acn3.51210.
8. Radmanesh A, Derman A, Lui YW, et al. COVID-19- associated diffuse leukoencephalopathy and microhemorrhages. Radiology. 2020;297(1):E223–7. https://doi.org/10.1148/radiol.2020202040.
9. Kantonen J, Mahzabin S, Mäyränpää MI, et al. Neuropathologic features of four autopsied COVID-19 patients. Brain Pathol. 2020;30(6):1012–6. https://doi.org/10.1111/bpa.12889.
10. Solomon IH, Normandin E, Bhattacharyya S, et al. Neuropathological features of Covid-19. N Engl J Med. 2020;383(10):989–92. https://doi.org/10.1056/NEJMc2019373.
11. Parsons T, Banks S, Bae C, et al. COVID-19- associated acute disseminated encephalomyelitis (ADEM). J Neurol. 2020;267(10):2799–802. https://doi.org/10.1007/s00415-020-09951-9.
12. Berlin DA, Gulick RM, Martinez FJ. Severe Covid-19. N Engl J Med. 2020;383(25):2451–60. https://doi.org/10.1056/NEJMcp2009575.

13. Connors JM, Levy JH. Thromboinflammation and the hypercoagulability of COVID-19. J Thromb Haemost. 2020;18(7):1559–61. https://doi.org/10.1111/jth.14849.
14. Shehata GA, Lord KC, Grudzinski MC, Elsayed M, Abdelnaby R, Elshabrawy HA. Neurological complications of COVID-19: underlying mechanisms and management. Int J Mol Sci. 2021;22:4081. https://doi.org/10.3390/ijms22084081.
15. Brundin P, Nath A, Beckham JD. Is COVID-19 a perfect storm for Parkinson's disease? Trends Neurosci. 2020;43(12):931–3. https://doi.org/10.1016/j.tins.2020.10.009.
16. Young MJ, O'Hare M, Matiello M, Schmahmann JD. Creutzfeldt-Jakob disease in a man with COVID-19: SARS-CoV-2-accelerated neurodegeneration? Brain Behav Immun. 2020;89:601–3. https://doi.org/10.1016/j.bbi.2020.07.007.
17. Zachariadis A, Tulbu A, Strambo D, et al. Transverse myelitis related to COVID-19 infection. J Neurol. 2020;267(12):3459–61. https://doi.org/10.1007/s00415-020-09997-9.
18. Toscano G, Palmerini F, Ravaglia S, et al. Guillain-Barré syndrome associated with SARS-CoV-2. N Engl J Med. 2020;382(26):2574–6. https://doi.org/10.1056/NEJMc2009191.
19. Zhang H, Charmchi Z, Seidman RJ, et al. COVID- 19-associated myositis with severe proximal and bulbar weakness. Muscle Nerve. 2020;62(3):E57–60. https://doi.org/10.1002/mus.27003.
20. Nath A. Long-haul COVID. Neurology. 2020;95(13):559–60. https://doi.org/10.1212/WNL.0000000000010640.

Psychiatric Issues After COVID-19

6

Gagan Hans and Rakesh Kumar Chadda

6.1 Introduction

The emergence of COVID-19 infection caused by SARS-CoV-2 is a catastrophic humanitarian crisis which may have widespread and long-lasting psychological effects [1]. It is expected that the resulting psychological distress experienced by different subgroups of the population is likely to be different based on their vulnerabilities. As the COVID-19 pandemic has progressed globally with repeated upsurges, the psychological impact has also been increasingly seen in vulnerable groups like healthcare workers, individuals in quarantine, and patients with chronic medical and psychiatric conditions [1]. Although the literature available on long-term impact is limited at present, there are preliminary indications that COVID-19 can produce long-term psychiatric sequelae.

6.2 Experiences from Past Coronavirus Outbreaks

Initially, the concerns regarding the psychiatric sequelae of the COVID-19 were based on the findings from outbreaks caused by other coronaviruses in the past [2]. It has been well documented that a patient with respiratory viral diseases can have both acute and long-term psychiatric sequelae [3]. There have been pandemics from other coronaviruses like SARS-CoV-1 in the past, for which the long-term effects on mental health have been well documented. Although extrapolation of these findings to the current situation is difficult, these can serve as useful

G. Hans (✉)
Department of Psychiatry, All India Institute of Medical Sciences, New Delhi, India

R. K. Chadda
Head, Department of Psychiatry and, Chief, National Drug Dependence Treatment Centre, All India Institute of Medical Sciences, New Delhi, India

A. Mohan, S. Mittal (eds.), *Post COVID-19 Complications and Management*,
https://doi.org/10.1007/978-981-19-4407-9_6

guiding principles for planning mental healthcare services. Psychiatric symptoms and disorders like post-traumatic stress disorder (PTSD) or its subsyndromal symptoms, anxiety, and depression have been documented in the patients, healthcare workers, and general population during previous coronavirus outbreaks, both at the time of pandemic and for variable durations afterward up to 3 years post-pandemic [4].

6.3 Mental Health Problems After COVID-19

Currently, published literature on the psychiatric sequelae in the post-COVID-19 illness phase is sparse, although insomnia, delirium, depression, anxiety, and PTSD have been commonly reported in the acute and convalescent phase [2]. A few studies have reported high rates of insomnia and symptoms of PTSD, anxiety, and depression after a duration of 1 month post-COVID-19 infection [5, 6]. There have also been suggestions that coronaviruses can lead to psychopathological sequelae either through direct infection of the central nervous system or indirectly mediated through the immune response it generates [7]. Coronaviruses are neurotropic, inducing neuronal injuries and leading to neuroinflammation, potentially causing neuropsychiatric manifestations [8, 9]. Also, studies have found that in addition to the increased risk of psychiatric outcomes associated with COVID-19 infection, the incidence was greater in patients who required hospitalization and significantly higher in patients requiring intensive care management [10]. The risk of having anxiety and depression remains consistently elevated even after 3–6 months of COVID-19 infection, and probably even beyond, along with an elevated risk of insomnia, psychosis, and substance use disorders [10]. Another large study found that a diagnosis of COVID-19 was associated with an increased incidence of having first psychiatric diagnosis within 14–90 days, especially for anxiety disorders, insomnia, and dementia. The same study also found that a psychiatric diagnosis in the previous year was independently associated with an increased incidence of COVID-19 diagnosis [11]. In addition, factors like poor socioeconomic status, loss of employment, limited access to essential supplies, special support needs, duration of lockdown, fear of infection, inadequate information, comorbid medical conditions, and advanced age could all be possible determinants of post-COVID-19 psychological sequelae [12].

Table 6.1 shows the high-risk groups for developing mental health problems post-COVID-19 pandemic.

The COVID-19 pandemic has resulted in employment losses for many workers in the private and unorganized sectors. Financial loss because of quarantine has been shown to produce negative psychological sequelae that can be long-lasting [13]. Evidence also suggests that the financial loss during quarantine can be a risk factor for subsequent development of symptoms of psychological disorders, [14] anger and anxiety [15], even months after the crisis is over. Financial and job losses in the post-COVID-19 period can also lead to an increase in the cases of domestic violence against women as the perpetual cycle of domestic violence is fuelled by

Table 6.1 High-risk groups for mental health problems post-COVID-19 pandemic

• Those with loss of immediate and long-term employment
• Women, children, and adolescents
• Senior citizens with/without special needs
• Homeless individuals with/without psychiatric illnesses, poor social support
• Lower socioeconomic status
• Persons with disabilities
• History of severe mental illness
• Frontline workers, including health professionals
• Life-threatening chronic medical conditions like cancer, chronic renal failure, liver diseases, asthma/chronic obstructive airway disease, immunocompromised individuals

factors such as low socioeconomic status, lesser wages, poor living conditions, a high number of children, ongoing pregnancy, alcohol, and other substance abuse [16]. This phenomenon has been described as a “pandemic within the pandemic.”

Children and adolescents have experienced disruptions in their regular schedules since schools and other everyday outdoor activities were suspended for a long time. This may result in various mental health issues, including anxiety, fear, worry, depression, difficulty sleeping, and appetite changes [17]. The experience of going through quarantine, isolation, or the death of a parent can further increase the chances of developing mental health issues in children and adolescents. Children with various physical and mental disabilities are especially vulnerable to developing these disorders as social isolation, economic hardships, and worsening physical and mental conditions of the parents and caregivers worsen the living condition of children with special needs or those living in abusive environments [17].

Elderly individuals, patients with chronic medical and psychiatric conditions, persons with disabilities, children, and other vulnerable subgroups are likely to depend on others for having an adequate basic supply of food, water, and other essentials. Having inadequate supplies of essentials can be a continued source of frustration [18] in the affected population and is persistently associated with anxiety and anger even at 4–6 months after quarantine [15]. These individuals, and patients suffering from chronic medical and psychiatric conditions, are also more likely to experience difficulties in their regular medical care, including getting prescriptions and regular supply of medications [18], compromising them further and leading to relapses of the medical and psychiatric disorders. Many people who are dependent on nicotine or alcohol or who have other psychoactive symptoms may experience acute withdrawal during the lockdown phase followed by worsening in the subsequent duration. There is also some evidence to suggest that a history of psychiatric illness is associated with persistent anxiety and anger even after 4–6 months post-infection [15].

Healthcare workers may experience high psychological distress during the pandemic, which increases the likelihood of developing post COVID-19 psychiatric sequelae. Poor working conditions combined with a lack of safety equipment and management protocol lead to increased chances of high-risk exposure necessitating quarantine, and/or getting infected. A history of quarantine in healthcare workers is

Table 6.2 Risk factors for developing anxiety and depression

• Living alone
• No children or ≥ 2 children
• Female gender
• Current medical/psychiatric illness
• Poor sleep quality
• Higher perceived stress
• Lacking knowledge of pandemic
• Impact on daily life
• Poor social support
• Impact on income
• Frontline workers

the most important predictor of developing acute stress disorder, PTSD, low mood, anger, exhaustion, anxiety, insomnia, irritability, poor concentration, decreased work performance, and reluctance to work or considering resignation [19, 20]. Quarantine also predisposes to development of PTSD and alcohol dependence in healthcare workers even after a long interval [20]. In addition, the severity of the symptoms of PTSD may be increased in the quarantined healthcare workers as compared to the quarantined individuals from the general population. They are also more likely to report greater stigma, loss of income, and avoidance behaviors in addition to greater fear, anger, frustration, sadness, worry, isolation, and helplessness post-quarantine. Healthcare workers are also likely to be more concerned about spreading the infection to their family members and to others in the surroundings [21]. There is emerging data to suggest that the healthcare professionals working in COVID-19 areas have significantly higher rates of depression, anxiety, and somatic symptoms than those working in non-COVID-19 areas in addition to the use of maladaptive coping strategies to cope with the resultant stress [22].

Table 6.2 enumerates several risk factors of developing anxiety and depression following COVID-19 infection [4].

6.4 Death, Dying, and Bereavement Issues

COVID-19 pandemic is expected to have a significant impact on the experience of death, dying, and bereavement. Studies from the previous pandemics have shown that a pandemic not only causes disruption directly due to death but also impacts and disrupts the social norms due to isolating measures, rituals, and mourning practices leading to potentially increased risk of developing complicated grief in the survivors [23]. The need for physical barriers and isolation measures, along with the use of personal protective equipment by family members and healthcare workers, limits the physical contact and number of visits from family members, causing loss of usual social support [24, 25]. Additionally, in case of loss due to death, the family members cannot support each other due to similar reasons [26]. During the pandemic, scarcity of hospital beds for admission also compromised the autonomy of the individuals regarding decisions about preferred place of death [26] and participation of others in decision-making process. Also, there was a disruption of the usual rituals and practices observed following death [27]. Thus, all these factors, along with the added risk of having multiple deaths in the same family, are likely to increase the risk of complicated grief in the survivors.

6.5 Prevention

To prevent the long-term impact of the pandemic, the resilience of the population is an important determinant. The resilience to the stress depends on several determinants, including socioeconomic condition, age, comorbid medical conditions, preexisting mental health conditions, length of the quarantine, food security, individual coping strategies, family support, and special needs [12]. Individually, establishing new routines, exercising regularly, and spending quality time with the family can help deal with the immediate stress and cope with the long-term effects of the pandemic. Judicious use of social media with information from reliable sources only can prevent information overload and avoid becoming overwhelmed with anxiety about the future course of events [12].

As multiple waves of the pandemic continue, the duration of the quarantine should be kept as minimum as possible based on the scientific reasoning of the incubation periods, as longer durations are associated with more negative psychological consequences [28]. Also, there should be provisions for free access to essential information regarding the pandemic through easily accessible means to prevent catastrophic appraisals by the affected individuals. Provisions for early identification of more vulnerable individuals like the elderly, people with high-risk comorbid medical conditions, and those with special needs can help in early treatment. Essential legislation and welfare schemes can protect the employment of the workers during lockdown period along with financial assistance. Similarly, assistance to seek work early in the post-COVID-19 phase can also help reduce the long-term psychological sequelae.

Healthcare workers should have clarity of their respective roles in the post-COVID-19 phase, including preparation for future waves of pandemic, and should be supported by means of adequate protective equipment and special accommodation near the workplace during the acute phase, which can alleviate their fear of spreading the infection to the family members. Legislation may be essential to protect the healthcare workers from stigmatizing attitudes in society. Organizational support is highly protective of mental health during infectious disease outbreaks, and staff should be supported in all possible ways to keep their morale high [29].

Telemedicine has emerged as an important vehicle of health services delivery in the COVID-19 pandemic. Telemedicine facilities should be encouraged, and helpline numbers should be established for people in distress as part of capacity building in the healthcare infrastructure. The release of telemedicine guidelines by the Board of Governors of Medical Council of India along with the release of

Telepsychiatry Operational Guidelines 2020 by the Indian Psychiatric Society, the Telemedicine Society of India, and the National Institute of Mental Health and Neurosciences has improved the horizons for mental healthcare in India during the COVID-19 pandemic. This should be further strengthened to improve mental health services provision in the post-pandemic phase [30].

6.6 Conclusions

In conclusion, the long-term psychological sequelae of COVID-19 are likely to pose a significant challenge and additional burden on already limited mental health services, especially in low- and middle-income countries. Measures like simple and precise information, minimum necessary lockdown period, adequate supply of essentials, protection of employment, and financial assistance to the poor will go a long way in minimizing these long-term adverse psychological effects. Technological advances in telemedicine have a key role to play in mental health services delivery in the foreseeable future.

6.7 Take-Home Messages

- Protection and special provisions for vulnerable groups, including healthcare workers, should be a priority to prevent long-term negative psychological effects.
- COVID-19 pandemic is expected to have a significant impact on the experience of death, dying, and bereavement resulting in increased risk of complicated grief.
- Measures like providing simple and clear public information, minimum necessary lockdown period, adequate supply of essentials, protection of employment, and financial assistance to those in need can help reduce long-term negative psychological effects.
- Long-term psychiatric sequelae are likely to put an additional burden on limited mental health resources in low- and middle-income countries.

References

1. Holmes EA, O'Connor RC, Perry VH, et al. Multidisciplinary research priorities for the COVID-19 pandemic: a call for action for mental health science. Lancet Psychiatry. 2020;7:547–60.
2. Rogers JP, Chesney E, Oliver D, et al. Psychiatric and neuropsychiatric presentations associated with severe coronavirus infections: a systematic review and meta-analysis with comparison to the COVID-19 pandemic. Lancet Psychiatry. 2020;7:611–27.
3. Bohmwald K, Galvez NMS, Rios M, et al. Neurologic alterations due to respiratory virus infections. Front Cell Neurosci. 2018;12:386.
4. Vindegaard N, Eriksen BM. COVID-19 pandemic and mental health consequences: systematic review of the current evidence. Brain Behav Immun. 2020;89:531–42.

5. Mazza MG, De Lorenzo R, Conte C, et al. Anxiety and depression in COVID-19 survivors: role of inflammatory and clinical predictors. Brain Behav Immun. 2020;89:594–600.
6. Tomasoni D, Bai F, Castoldi R, et al. Anxiety and depression symptoms after virological clearance of COVID-19: a cross-sectional study in Milan. Italy J Med Virol. 2021;93:1175–9.
7. Wu Y, Xu X, Chen Z, et al. Nervous system involvement after infection with COVID-19 and other coronaviruses. Brain Behav Immun. 2020;87:18–22.
8. Dantzer R. Neuroimmune interactions: from the brain to the immune system and vice versa. Physiol Rev. 2018;98:477–504.
9. Desforges M, Le Coupanec A, Dubeau P, et al. Human coronaviruses and other respiratory viruses: underestimated opportunistic pathogens of the central nervous system? Viruses. 2019;12(1):14.
10. Taquet M, Geddes JR, Husain M, et al. 6-month neurological and psychiatric outcomes in 236379 survivors of COVID-19: a retrospective cohort study using electronic health records. Lancet Psychiatry. 2021;8(5):416–27.
11. Taquet M, Luciano S, Geddes JR, et al. Bidirectional associations between COVID-19 and psychiatric disorder: retrospective cohort studies of 62354 COVID-19 cases in the USA. Lancet Psychiatry. 2021;8:130–40.
12. Hans G, Gupte N, Faheem A, et al. Acute psychological effects in the times of COVID-19 pandemic. Delhi Ophthalmology Society Times, COVID-19 Special. 2020;25(4):65–8.
13. Brooks SK, Webster RK, Smith LE, et al. The psychological impact of quarantine and how to reduce it: rapid review of the evidence. Lancet. 2020;395:912–20.
14. Mihashi M, Otsubo Y, Yinjuan X, et al. Predictive factors of psychological disorder development during recovery following SARS outbreak. Health Psychol. 2009;28:91–100.
15. Jeong H, Yim HW, Song Y-J, et al. Mental health status of people isolated due to Middle East respiratory syndrome. Epidemiol Health. 2016;38:e2016048.
16. Sagar R, Hans G. Domestic violence and mental health. J Mental Health Hum Behav. 2018;23:2–3.
17. Mental Health Assessment of COVID-19 Patient in Health Care & Community Settings; Mental Health in the times of COVID-19 Pandemic Guidance for General Medical and Specialised Mental Health Care Settings, April 2020, 18-24. Available at https://nimhans.ac.in/wp-content/uploads/2020/04/MentalHealthIssuesCOVID-19NIMHANS.pdf. Last accessed November 14, 2021.
18. Blendon RJ, Benson JM, DesRoches CM, et al. The public's response to severe acute respiratory syndrome in Toronto and the United States. Clin Infect Dis. 2004;38:925–31.
19. Bai Y, Lin C-C, Lin C-Y, et al. Survey of stress reactions among health care workers involved with the SARS outbreak. Psychiatr Serv. 2004;55:1055–7.
20. Wu P, Fang Y, Guan Z, et al. The psychological impact of the SARS epidemic on hospital employees in China: exposure, risk perception, and altruistic acceptance of risk. Can J Psychiatr. 2009;54:302–11.
21. Reynolds DL, Garay JR, Deamond SL, et al. Understanding, compliance and psychological impact of the SARS quarantine experience. Epidemiol Infect. 2008;136:997–1007.
22. Singh J, Sood M, Chadda RK, et al. Mental health issues and coping among health care workers during COVID19 pandemic. Indian perspective. Asian J Psychiatr. 2021;61:102685.
23. Mayland CR, Harding AJ, Preston N, et al. Supporting adults bereaved through COVID-19: a rapid review of the impact of previous pandemics on grief and bereavement. J Pain Symptom Manag. 2020;60(2):e33–9.
24. Rabelo I, Lee V, Fallah MP, et al. Psychological distress among Ebola survivors discharged from an Ebola treatment unit in Monrovia, Liberia e a qualitative study. Front Public Health. 2016;4:142.
25. Schwerdtle PM, De Clerck V, Plummer V. Experience of Ebola survivors: causes of distress and sources of resilience. Prehosp Disaster Med. 2017;32:234–9.
26. Leong IY, Lee AO, Ng TW, et al. The challenges of providing holistic care in a viral epidemic: opportunities for palliative care. Pall Med. 2004;18:12–8.

27. Grimaud J, Legahneur F. Community beliefs and fears during a cholera outbreak in Haiti. Intervention. 2011;9:26–34.
28. Hawryluck L, Gold WL, Robinson S, et al. SARS control and psychological effects of quarantine, Toronto, Canada. Emerg Infect Dis. 2004;10:1206–12.
29. Brooks SK, Dunn R, Amlôt R, et al. A systematic, thematic review of social and occupational factors associated with psychological outcomes in healthcare employees during an infectious disease outbreak. J Occup Environ Med. 2018;60:248–57.
30. Kumari R, Padhy SK, Chadda RK, et al. The Telepsychiatry operational guidelines 2020 in India: a welcome step. BJPsych Int. 2021;18(4):e12,1.

Long-term Gastrointestinal Complications Following COVID-19

7

Anshuman Elhence and Uday C. Ghoshal

7.1 Introduction

It has been over 2 years since the severe acute respiratory syndrome coronavirus 2 (SARS- CoV-2), a beta coronavirus, spread from Wuhan city in the Hubei province of China to evolve into a pandemic of coronavirus disease 2019 (COVID-19) affecting the whole world [1]. Despite widespread vaccination and healthcare infrastructure upscaling, the pandemic has been difficult to control due to emerging variants of concern (VOC) such as the delta and omicron variants which continue to cause staggering waves of the pandemic.

The virus, SARS-CoV-2, is a single-stranded ribonucleic acid (RNA) virus which has tropism for the respiratory system which explains its nomenclature. The viral nucleic acid codes for four different proteins include the spike (S), envelope (E), membrane (M), and nucleocapsid (N) proteins [2]. The viral S protein utilizes the angiotensin-converting enzyme-2 (ACE-2) receptor, a host metallopeptidase, to enter the host cell [3]. Another host protease, the transmembrane serine protease (TMPRSS 2 and 4), helps in cleavage of the viral S protein and facilitation of internalization of the virus inside host cells [4]. Due to the widespread expression of ACE-2 receptor on the nasal, nasopharyngeal, and respiratory tract mucosa, COVID-19 presents in majority with fever and upper respiratory tract symptoms such as cough and coryza [3]. However, in a minority of patients, particularly those with comorbid illness such as diabetes, obesity, cardiopulmonary illness, chronic kidney, and liver disease, it may take the form of a life-threatening severe acute respiratory syndrome [5].

Since, the ACE-2 receptor is expressed widely throughout the gastrointestinal tract including the esophagus, stomach, small and large intestine, liver, and

A. Elhence · U. C. Ghoshal (✉)
Department of Gastroenterology, Sanjay Gandhi Post Graduate Institute of Medical Sciences, Lucknow, India

A. Mohan, S. Mittal (eds.), *Post COVID-19 Complications and Management*, https://doi.org/10.1007/978-981-19-4407-9_7

pancreas, not surprisingly gastrointestinal manifestations are not uncommon [3]. A systematic review and meta-analysis of 60 studies with over 4000 patients showed that gastrointestinal symptoms are present in up to one-fifth of patients and nearly half of patients excrete the SARS-CoV-2 in feces even after testing negative from nasopharyngeal samples [6]. The prevalence of gastrointestinal symptoms particularly diarrhea, nausea, and stool urgency has been found to be as high as 60%, and nausea has been shown to persist beyond 1 month on follow-up [7]. Besides the gastrointestinal tract proper, COVID-19 has been shown to cause alteration in liver function tests in up to 50% of patients and affect the pancreas in a minority [8, 9]. The gastrointestinal manifestations of COVID-19 are important to recognize, not only because of concern for feco-oral transmission of the virus apart from the well-recognized droplet route but also because a subset of patients (5%) may present with only gastrointestinal symptoms and hence may escape detection in absence of a high degree of suspicion [10].

As our experience with COVID-19 grows, reports of new-onset or prolonged neuromuscular, respiratory, and gastrointestinal symptoms persisting after recovery from COVID-19, termed the post-COVID-19 syndrome or "long-haul" COVID-19, are emerging [11]. In this chapter we explore the pathogenesis, epidemiology, and management of post-COVID-19 gastrointestinal manifestations.

7.2 Pathophysiological Mechanisms

With the emerging information on COVID-19, there are some mechanistic insights into the pathophysiology behind acute gastrointestinal symptoms of COVID-19 [12]. However, the long-term sequelae remain an enigma with limited information into its mechanisms. The exact mechanisms underlying the development of functional gastrointestinal disorders (FGIDs) are not well known. However, there is some evidence for a microorganic basis for these disorders which is best exemplified by post-infection (PI)-FGIDs (Fig. 7.1).

7.2.1 Concept of Post-Infection Disorders of Gut-Brain Interaction

Following bacterial, viral, or protozoal infections, PI-FGIDs, which now have been more appropriately rechristened as disorders of gut-brain interaction (DGBI), are common and develop in nearly 11% of the patients [13]. Although classically described to develop as a sequelae of invasive bacterial gastroenteritis, of late they have been found to develop following viral gastroenteritis as well, albeit at a lower frequency (Table 7.1) [14–17]. These FGIDs encompass the spectrum of irritable bowel syndrome (IBS), commonly diarrhea predominant (IBS-D) as well as

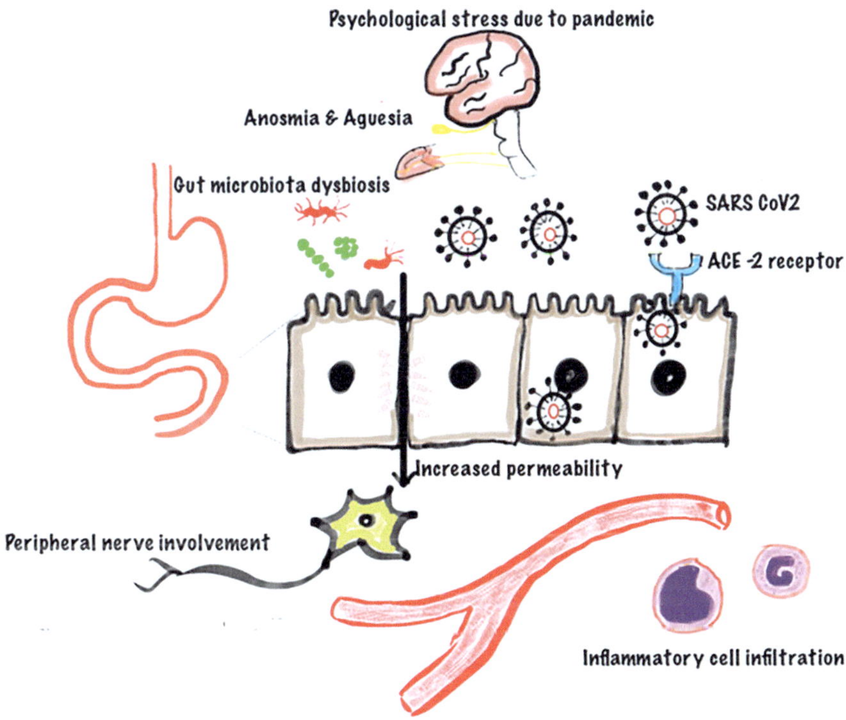

Fig. 7.1 Purported mechanisms underlying long-term gastrointestinal manifestation of COVID-19

functional dyspepsia (FD) [18]. Since COVID-19 is well known to cause gastrointestinal symptoms, a definition of post-COVID-19 FGID has been proposed when this symptom complex meeting the established criteria of FGIDs develops after a documented SARS-CoV-2 infection [12, 19].

7.2.2 ACE-2-Mediated Mechanisms

The ACE-2, via its role in the renin-angiotensin system (RAS) has been linked to regulation of intestinal blood flow, permeability, motility, and fluid and electrolyte absorption [20]. Deficiency of ACE-2 has been shown to predispose to inflammation and colitis in murine models [21]. It has been hypothesized that the gastrointestinal symptoms may arise due to the direct effect of the virus on the receptor leading to alteration of its functions or a secondary downregulation of ACE-2 as a result of SARS-CoV-2 infection [12]

Table 7.1 Studies on post-viral functional gastrointestinal diseases

Author	Journal	Year	Country	Virus	Risk	Comments
Marshall et al.	CGH	2007	Canada	Norovirus	OR 6.9 (1.0–48.8)	–
Zanini et al.	AJG	2012	Italy	Norovirus	OR 11.4 (3.4–37.8)	–
Saps et al.	JPGN	2009	Italy and USA	Rotavirus	7/44 (16%) in cases vs 3/44 (7%) in controls	Pediatric study
Porter et al.	CID	2012	USA	Norovirus	IBS OR 0.68 (0.3–1.52) Dyspepsia OR 1.44 (0.84–2.47)	Only negative study for IBS
Ghoshal et al.	JGH	2021	India, Bangladesh	SARS-CoV2	IBS 15 (5.3%), Dyspepsia 6 (2.1%), Overlap 5(1.8%) in cases vs IBS 1 (0.4%) in control at 6 months	

Abbreviations: *CGH* Clinical Gastroenterology and Hepatology; *OR* odds ratio; *AJG* American Journal of Gastroenterology; *JPGN* Journal of Pediatric Gastroenterology and Nutrition; *USA* United States of America; *CID* Clinical Infectious Diseases; *IBS* Irritable bowel syndrome; *JGH* Journal of Gastroenterology and Hepatology; *SARS-CoV2* Severe acute respiratory syndrome coronavirus 2

7.2.3 Persistent Intestinal Inflammation

Once the SARS-CoV-2 infects the enterocytes, it evokes an inflammatory response which has not been well characterized but is accompanied by infiltration of the mucosa with neutrophils, macrophages, and lymphocytes. Fecal calprotectin (FCP), an inflammatory marker released by neutrophils, not only has been found to be raised among those with COVID-19 as compared to controls, but also is higher among those with diarrhea as compared to without diarrhea [22–24]. This increase in FCP has been shown to persist even after resolution of diarrhea, and the FCP levels have been shown to correlate with interleukin-6 (IL-6) levels [22]. Moreover, higher levels of pro-inflammatory cytokines (IL-8, IL-23) and lower levels of anti-inflammatory cytokines (IL-10) have been demonstrated in the feces of patients with COVID-19 as compared to controls hinting toward intestinal inflammation caused by the virus. The intestinal inflammation induced by the virus has been demonstrated by histopathology as infiltration of the lamina propria in the stomach, small bowel, and colon with mononuclear inflammatory cells [25].

7.2.4 Gut Microbiota Dysbiosis

It has been shown that even among antibiotic-naïve COVID-19 patients, the delicate balance of gut microbes is disrupted by SARS-CoV-2 and is characterized by decrease in symbionts such as *Faecalibacterium prausnitzii*, *Eubacterium ventriosum*, *Roseburia*, and Lachnospiraceae and increase in opportunistic microbes such as *Clostridium hathewayi*, *Bacteroides nordi*, and *Actinomyces viscosus* [26]. In fact, baseline abundance of certain species such as *Coprobacillus*, *Clostridium ramosum*, and *Clostridium hathewayi* correlated directly with COVID-19 severity, while that of *Faecalibacterium prausnitzii* correlated inversely with severity of COVID-19 [26]. These changes in gut microbiota have been shown to persist beyond hospital discharge [27]. The functional profile of this altered microbiome is characterized by depletion of short-chain fatty acids (SCFAs) which have a well-known anti-inflammatory role as well as a role in downregulation of the ACE-2 receptor and hence possibly COVID-19 severity [27, 28]. The development of PI-FGIDs has been strongly linked to gut dysbiosis, and hence it has been hypothesized that such a post-COVID-19 dysbiosis may contribute toward the prolonged gastrointestinal symptoms.

7.2.5 Altered Serotonergic Signaling

Serotonin (5-hydroxy tryptamine [5-HT]) is secreted by the enterochromaffin cells in the gastrointestinal tract in response to a variety of mechanical and chemical stimuli and in turn acts as a neurocrine and paracrine signaling agent regulating a variety of sensory, motor, and secretory functions [29]. In fact, altered serotonergic signaling has been demonstrated in a number of FGIDs [30]. A number of pharmacological agents such as 5-HT3 antagonists to treat IBS-D (e.g., ramosetron, alosetron) and 5-HT4 agonists to treat IBS-constipation predominant (IBS-C) such as cisapride and tegaserod are testimony to the disordered serotonergic signaling in IBS. Higher levels of 5-HT have been shown in patients with COVID-19-associated diarrhea as compared to COVID-19 patients without diarrhea as well as healthy controls and may play a role in the persistent gastrointestinal symptoms after recovery from COVID-19 [31].

7.2.6 Altered Gastrointestinal Permeability

The tight junction proteins including occludin, claudin, and junctional adhesion molecules regulate intestinal permeability via the paracellular pathway and are under the influence of a number of physiological stimuli as well as pathological stressors [29]. Altered intestinal mucosal permeability has been demonstrated in COVID-19 patients [32]. It has been hypothesized that altered permeability leads to an aberrant mucosal immune response which may contribute to FGID symptoms [29].

7.2.7 Involvement of Central and Peripheral Nervous System

Central hypervigilance and psychological comorbidities such as anxiety, depression, stress, and hypochondriasis are well-known risk factors for PI-IBS [13]. The pandemic has brought with it a sense of fear, apprehension of infection, as well as post-traumatic stress disorders among survivors and those who have suffered loss of family members [33, 34]. Moreover, the SARS-CoV-2 has been shown to involve the central nervous system directly as evidenced by inflammation of the olfactory bulb, cerebrum, and brainstem [35, 36]. Not surprisingly, anosmia and ageusia which arise due to involvement of olfactory bulb and facial and glossopharyngeal cranial nerves, respectively, found in up to a quarter of patients with COVID-19 have been found to be associated with development of post-COVID-19 FGID [37].

7.3 Prevalence and Spectrum

As the pandemic is progressing and there is an ever-increasing pool of post-COVID-19 survivors, our knowledge about the post-COVID-19 gastrointestinal sequelae is also increasing.

It has been recently shown in a multicentric case-control study from our group that at 6 months following COVID-19, IBS, dyspepsia, and their overlap develop in 5.3%, 2.1%, and 1.8% patients, respectively [37]. Presence of anosmia, ageusia, chronic bowel dysfunction, and dyspepsia at 1 and 3 months and psychological comorbidity were predictors for development of post-COVID-19 FGID [37]. A few other studies have tried exploring the long-term gastrointestinal manifestations following COVID-19 (Table 7.2) [38–40]. In a telephonic survey of post-COVID-19 ambulatory patients 6 months after recovery, Velez et al. showed that nearly 40% of them developed de novo gastrointestinal symptoms [40]. Of the 200 patients followed up, 79 had post-COVID-19 gastrointestinal symptoms with the majority having dyspepsia (29%), IBS-like symptoms (1%), and their overlap (10%) [40]. Female gender, presence of anxiety and depression, and gastrointestinal symptoms at the time of COVID-19 were associated with development of these sequelae [40]. In another online case-control survey of COVID-19 patients and controls done 5 months post-recovery, the prevalence of Rome IV-defined IBS was similar between cases and controls (26% vs 25%, $p = 0.81$); however loose stools (Bristol ≥6) were more common in post-COVID-19 group (18% vs 9%, $p = 0.02$) as compared to controls [38]. Other studies evaluating long-term gastrointestinal symptoms have also shown that close to 5%–10% of patients often have persistent symptoms in form of abdominal pain, constipation, diarrhea, and nausea at long-term follow-up [39].

There is limited mechanistic insight into the mechanisms of these symptoms; however mechanisms similar to PI-IBS have been invoked as discussed above.

Table 7.2 Studies on long-term gastrointestinal manifestations of COVID-19

Author	Journal, Year	Country	Study design	Sample size	Follow-up duration	Comments
Ghoshal et al	JGH, 2021	India, Bangladesh	Case-control	Cases: 280 Controls: 264	6 months	First controlled study to use formal Rome-criteria
Blackett et al	NGM, 2021	USA	Retrospective, Observational	147	106 days	Abdominal pain (7.5%) was most common sequelae followed by constipation (6.8%)
Noviello et al	NGM, 2021	Italy	Case-control	Cases: 164 Controls: 183	5 months	IBS (Rome IV) was similar between cases and controls
Velez et al	CGH, 2021	USA	Retrospective, observational	200	6 months	40% patients had new onset symptoms. Limitation: Performed over telephonic survey with monetary renumeration

Abbreviations: *COVID-19* coronavirus disease; *JGH* Journal of Gastroenterology and Hepatology; *NGM* Neurogastroenterology and motility; *CGH* Clinical Gastroenterology and Hepatology; *USA* United States of America

7.4 Management

Since data on the spectrum and mechanisms underlying the long-term gastrointestinal sequelae are still emerging, there is limited insight of appropriate treatment options. However, the treatment principles have largely been borrowed from PI-IBS. Opiates (loperamide, diphenoxylate, and eluxadoline), 5-HT3 receptor antagonists (ramosetron, ondansetron, and alosetron), bile acid modulators (cholestyramine, colestipol, and colesevelam), rifaximin, probiotics (*Saccharomyces boulardii*, *Lactobacillus*), and fiber supplements (polycarbophil and psyllium) have been used empirically as for IBS-D [13]. Although 5-aminosalicylic acid (5-ASA) and glutamine have specifically shown benefit in PI-IBS, either is yet to be tested in patients with post-COVID-19 IBS-like symptoms [41, 42]. Visceral neuromodulators like tricyclic antidepressants are often used to treat FGIDs because apart from their central action, the anticholinergic activity helps decrease diarrhea [13].

7.5 Conclusion

Long-term sequelae of SARS-CoV-2 infection may persist even after recovery from COVID-19. The post COVID-19 symptom complex includes a myriad of symptoms including persistent fatigue, brain fog, myalgia, respiratory symptoms, and gastrointestinal symptoms, termed "long COVID" or "long-haul COVID-19." Gastrointestinal symptoms in form of abdominal pain, diarrhea, constipation, dyspepsia, or a combination thereof may persist in 5%–10% of patients. These may take the form of well-defined FGIDs like IBS and FD. Currently there is limited information about the underlying mechanisms and treatment options. However, it is hypothesized that these might be similar to post-infection FGIDs.

Financial Disclosures None.

Conflict of Interest None.

References

1. Zhou P, Yang X-L, Wang X-G, Hu B, Zhang L, Zhang W, et al. A pneumonia outbreak associated with a new coronavirus of probable bat origin. Nature. 2020 Mar;579(7798):270–3.
2. Ghoshal UC, Ghoshal U, Dhiman RK. Gastrointestinal and hepatic involvement in severe acute respiratory syndrome coronavirus 2 infection: a review. J Clin Exp Hepatol. 2020;10(6):622–8.
3. Hamming I, Timens W, Bulthuis MLC, Lely AT, Navis GJ, van Goor H. Tissue distribution of ACE2 protein, the functional receptor for SARS coronavirus. A first step in understanding SARS pathogenesis. J Pathol. 2004 Jun;203(2):631–7.
4. Zang R, Gomez Castro MF, McCune BT, Zeng Q, Rothlauf PW, Sonnek NM, et al. TMPRSS2 and TMPRSS4 promote SARS-CoV-2 infection of human small intestinal enterocytes. Sci Immunol. 2020 May 13;5(47):eabc3582.
5. Elhence A, Shalimar. COVID-19: beyond respiratory tract. J Dig Endosc. 2020;11(1):24–6.
6. Cheung KS, Hung IFN, Chan PPY, Lung KC, Tso E, Liu R, et al. Gastrointestinal manifestations of SARS-CoV-2 infection and virus load in fecal samples from a Hong Kong cohort: systematic review and meta-analysis. Gastroenterology. 2020 Jul;159(1):81–95.
7. Marasco G, Cremon C, Barbaro MR, Salvi D, Cacciari G, Kagramanova A, et al. Prevalence of gastrointestinal symptoms in severe acute respiratory syndrome coronavirus 2 infection: results of the prospective controlled multinational GI-COVID-19 study. Am J Gastroenterol. 2022 Jan 1;117(1):147–57.
8. Elhence A, Vaishnav M, Biswas S, Chauhan A, Anand A, Shalimar. Coronavirus Disease-2019 (COVID-19) and the liver. J Clin Transl Hepatol. 2021 Apr 28;9(2):247–55.
9. Samanta J, Mahapatra SJ, Kumar N, Elhence A, Dhar J, Gupta A, et al. Virus induced acute pancreatitis and virus superinfection in the 'dual disease' model of acute pancreatitis and SARS-co-V2 infection: a multicentre prospective study. Pancreatology [Internet] 2022 Jan 25 [cited 2022 Jan 26]; Available from: https://www.sciencedirect.com/science/article/pii/S1424390322000096
10. Ghoshal UC, Ghoshal U, Mathur A, Singh RK, Nath A, Garg A, et al. The Spectrum of gastrointestinal symptoms in patients with coronavirus Disease-19: predictors, relationship with disease severity, and outcome. Clin Transl Gastroenterol. 2020 Nov 20;11(12):e00259.

11. Nalbandian A, Sehgal K, Gupta A, Madhavan MV, McGroder C, Stevens JS, et al. Post-acute COVID-19 syndrome. Nat Med. 2021 Apr;27(4):601–15.
12. Settanni CR, Ianiro G, Ponziani FR, Bibbò S, Segal JP, Cammarota G, et al. COVID-19 as a trigger of irritable bowel syndrome: a review of potential mechanisms. World J Gastroenterol. 2021 Nov 21;27(43):7433–45.
13. Ghoshal UC. Postinfection Irritable Bowel Syndrome. Gut Liver [Internet]. [cited 2022 Jan 26]; Available from: https://www.gutnliver.org/journal/view.html?doi=10.5009/gnl210208
14. Marshall JK, Thabane M, Borgaonkar MR, James C. Postinfectious irritable bowel syndrome after a food-borne outbreak of acute gastroenteritis attributed to a viral pathogen. Clin Gastroenterol Hepatol Off Clin Pract J Am Gastroenterol Assoc. 2007 Apr;5(4):457–60.
15. Zanini B, Ricci C, Bandera F, Caselani F, Magni A, Laronga AM, et al. Incidence of post-infectious irritable bowel syndrome and functional intestinal disorders following a water-borne viral gastroenteritis outbreak. Am J Gastroenterol. 2012 Jun;107(6):891–9.
16. Saps M, Pensabene L, Turco R, Staiano A, Cupuro D, Di Lorenzo C. Rotavirus gastroenteritis: precursor of functional gastrointestinal disorders? J Pediatr Gastroenterol Nutr. 2009 Nov;49(5):580–3.
17. Porter CK, Faix DJ, Shiau D, Espiritu J, Espinosa BJ, Riddle MS. Postinfectious gastrointestinal disorders following norovirus outbreaks. Clin Infect Dis Off Publ Infect Dis Soc Am. 2012 Oct;55(7):915–22.
18. Ford AC, Thabane M, Collins SM, Moayyedi P, Garg AX, Clark WF, et al. Prevalence of uninvestigated dyspepsia 8 years after a large waterborne outbreak of bacterial dysentery: a cohort study. Gastroenterology. 2010 May;138(5):1727–36.
19. Schmulson M, Ghoshal UC, Barbara G. Managing the inevitable surge of post-COVID-19 functional gastrointestinal disorders. Am J Gastroenterol. 2021 Jan 1;116(1):4–7.
20. Fändriks L. The angiotensin II type 2 receptor and the gastrointestinal tract. J Renin-Angiotensin-Aldosterone Syst JRAAS. 2010 Mar;11(1):43–8.
21. Hashimoto T, Perlot T, Rehman A, Trichereau J, Ishiguro H, Paolino M, et al. ACE2 links amino acid malnutrition to microbial ecology and intestinal inflammation. Nature. 2012 Jul 25;487(7408):477–81.
22. Effenberger M, Grabherr F, Mayr L, Schwaerzler J, Nairz M, Seifert M, et al. Faecal calprotectin indicates intestinal inflammation in COVID-19. Gut. 2020 Aug;69(8):1543–4.
23. Britton GJ, Chen-Liaw A, Cossarini F, Livanos AE, Spindler MP, Plitt T, et al. Limited intestinal inflammation despite diarrhea, fecal viral RNA and SARS-CoV-2-specific IgA in patients with acute COVID-19. Sci Rep. 2021 Jun 25;11(1):13308.
24. Jena A, Kumar-M P, Singh AK, Sharma V. Fecal calprotectin levels in COVID-19: lessons from a systematic review on its use in inflammatory bowel disease during the pandemic. Dig Liver Dis Off J Ital Soc Gastroenterol Ital Assoc Study Liver. 2021 Mar;53(3):295–7.
25. Deshmukh V, Motwani R, Kumar A, Kumari C, Raza K. Histopathological observations in COVID-19: a systematic review. J Clin Pathol. 2021 Feb;74(2):76–83.
26. Zuo T, Zhang F, Lui GCY, Yeoh YK, Li AYL, Zhan H, et al. Alterations in gut microbiota of patients with COVID-19 during time of hospitalization. Gastroenterology. 2020 Sep;159(3):944–955.e8.
27. Zhang F, Wan Y, Zuo T, Yeoh YK, Liu Q, Zhang L, et al. Prolonged impairment of short-chain fatty acid and L-isoleucine biosynthesis in gut microbiome in patients with COVID-19. Gastroenterology. 2022 Feb;162(2):548–561.e4.
28. Li J, Richards EM, Handberg EM, Pepine CJ, Raizada MK. Butyrate regulates COVID-19–relevant genes in gut epithelial organoids from normotensive rats. Hypertension. 2021 Feb 1;77(2):e13–6.
29. Barbara G, Feinle-Bisset C, Ghoshal UC, Quigley EM, Santos J, Vanner S, et al. The intestinal microenvironment and functional gastrointestinal disorders. Gastroenterology. 2016 Feb 18;S0016-5085(16):00219–5.
30. Kumar S, Ranjan P, Mittal B, Ghoshal UC. Serotonin transporter gene (SLC6A4) polymorphism in patients with irritable bowel syndrome and healthy controls. J Gastrointest Liver Dis JGLD. 2012 Mar;21(1):31–8.

31. Ha S, Jin B, Clemmensen B, Park P, Mahboob S, Gladwill V, et al. Serotonin is elevated in COVID-19-associated diarrhoea. Gut. 2021 Oct;70(10):2015–7.
32. Cardinale V, Capurso G, Ianiro G, Gasbarrini A, Arcidiacono PG, Alvaro D. Intestinal permeability changes with bacterial translocation as key events modulating systemic host immune response to SARS-CoV-2: a working hypothesis. Dig Liver Dis. 2020 Dec;52(12):1383–9.
33. Mazza MG, De Lorenzo R, Conte C, Poletti S, Vai B, Bollettini I, et al. Anxiety and depression in COVID-19 survivors: role of inflammatory and clinical predictors. Brain Behav Immun. 2020 Oct;89:594–600.
34. Santomauro DF, Herrera AMM, Shadid J, Zheng P, Ashbaugh C, Pigott DM, et al. Global prevalence and burden of depressive and anxiety disorders in 204 countries and territories in 2020 due to the COVID-19 pandemic. Lancet. 2021 Nov 6;398(10312):1700–12.
35. Reza-Zaldívar EE, Hernández-Sapiéns MA, Minjarez B, Gómez-Pinedo U, Márquez-Aguirre AL, Mateos-Díaz JC, et al. Infection mechanism of SARS-COV-2 and its implication on the nervous system. Front Immunol. 2020;11:621735.
36. Schurink B, Roos E, Radonic T, Barbe E, Bouman CSC, de Boer HH, et al. Viral presence and immunopathology in patients with lethal COVID-19: a prospective autopsy cohort study. Lancet Microbe. 2020 Nov 1;1(7):e290–9.
37. Ghoshal UC, Ghoshal U, Rahman MM, Mathur A, Rai S, Akhter M, et al. Post-infection functional gastrointestinal disorders following coronavirus disease-19: a case–control study. J Gastroenterol Hepatol. 2021 Nov 4; https://doi.org/10.1111/jgh.15717.
38. Noviello D, Costantino A, Muscatello A, Bandera A, Consonni D, Vecchi M, et al. Functional gastrointestinal and somatoform symptoms five months after SARS-CoV-2 infection: a controlled cohort study. Neurogastroenterol Motil. n/a(n/a):e14187.
39. Blackett JW, Li J, Jodorkovsky D, Freedberg DE. Prevalence and risk factors for gastrointestinal symptoms after recovery from COVID-19. Neurogastroenterol Motil Off J Eur Gastrointest Motil Soc. 2021 Sep;1:e14251.
40. Vélez C, Paz M, Silvernale C, Stratton LW, Kuo B, Staller K, et al. Factors associated with chronic De novo post-coronavirus disease gastrointestinal disorders in a metropolitan US County. Clin Gastroenterol Hepatol [Internet] 2021 Oct 21 [cited 2022 Jan 26]; Available from: https://www.sciencedirect.com/science/article/pii/S1542356521011332
41. Zhou Q, Verne ML, Fields JZ, Lefante JJ, Basra S, Salameh H, et al. Randomised placebo-controlled trial of dietary glutamine supplements for postinfectious irritable bowel syndrome. Gut. 2019 Jun;68(6):996–1002.
42. Lam C, Tan W, Leighton M, Hastings M, Lingaya M, Falcone Y, et al. A mechanistic multicentre, parallel group, randomised placebo-controlled trial of mesalazine for the treatment of IBS with diarrhoea (IBS-D). Gut. 2016 Jan;65(1):91–9.

Post-COVID-19 Endocrine Abnormalities

8

Alpesh Goyal and Nikhil Tandon

8.1 Introduction

The coronavirus disease 2019 (COVID-19) pandemic caused by severe acute respiratory syndrome coronavirus 2 (SARS-CoV-2) has emerged as a global health challenge. The SARS-CoV-2 uses angiotensin-converting enzyme 2 (ACE2) as the receptor to gain entry into host cells [1]. The disease manifestations, both during the acute and post-acute phase, may extend beyond the respiratory system and involve other systems, including the endocrine system (Table 8.1). The ACE2 receptor is expressed by endocrine organs, including the hypothalamus and pituitary, thyroid, pancreas, adrenals, and testes, and may result in direct gland damage [2]. Furthermore, the immunological cascade triggered by the hyper-inflammatory state of infection may trigger autoimmunity in predisposed individuals [3]. SARS-CoV-2 vaccines, including inactivated whole-virion, viral vector, and mRNA vaccines, have also been reported to cause endocrine adverse events (Table 8.1). In this chapter, we discuss post-acute phase endocrine complications of SARS-CoV-2 infection/vaccines and their mechanisms, emphasizing the need for increased awareness and close clinical surveillance to improve patient outcomes.

A. Goyal · N. Tandon (✉)
Department of Endocrinology and Metabolism, All India Institute of Medical Sciences, New Delhi, India

A. Mohan, S. Mittal (eds.), *Post COVID-19 Complications and Management*,
https://doi.org/10.1007/978-981-19-4407-9_8

Table 8.1 Endocrine complications reported following SARS-CoV-2 infection and vaccination

Hypothalamus and pituitary
• Hypophysitis (following infection and vaccine, both) • Isolated central diabetes insipidus • Isolated central hypocortisolism • Pituitary apoplexy
Thyroid
• Subacute thyroiditis (following infection and vaccine, both) • Graves' disease (following infection and vaccine, both)
Pancreas
• New-onset diabetes
Adrenal
• Adrenal hemorrhage and primary adrenal insufficiency (following infection and vaccine, both) • Autoimmune adrenal insufficiency
Gonads
• Low serum testosterone • Sertoli cell dysfunction and disruption of spermatogenesis

8.2 Hypothalamus and Pituitary Involvement

Hypothalamus and pituitary cells express ACE2 and are therefore potential targets for SARS-CoV-2. In the previous SARS outbreak, Leow et al. reported SARS-associated pituitary dysfunction in a cohort of 61 participants at 3 months following recovery from infection [4]. The pituitary dysfunction was related to either hypophysitis or direct hypothalamic involvement and involved the hypothalamic-pituitary-adrenal axis (24/61, 39%) more often compared to hypothalamic-pituitary-thyroid axis (3/61, 4.9%). Wheatland proposed that both SARS and influenza viruses use molecular mimicry of adrenocorticotrophic hormone (ACTH) as an immunoevasive strategy to blunt host stress response (through anti-ACTH antibodies) and thus create a state of relative adrenocortical insufficiency [5]. However, molecular mimicry of SARS-CoV-2 and ACTH has not been reported yet.

During the acute phase of SARS-CoV-2 infection, hyperprolactinemia, hyponatremia related to the syndrome of inappropriate antidiuretic hormone (SIADH) secretion, and pituitary apoplexy have been noted [2, 6]. On the other hand, hypophysitis, isolated pituitary hormone deficiency, and apoplexy can occur after recovery from COVID-19 or after SARS-CoV-2 vaccination (Table 8.2). Nonglait et al. reported lymphocytic adenohypophysitis in a 27-year-old male who presented 2 weeks following mild COVID-19 with hyponatremia and multiple anterior pituitary hormone deficits [7]. Although the authors did not perform a pituitary biopsy, the temporality of events and a known relationship between SARS-CoV-2 and pituitary suggest that hypophysitis was related to the viral infection itself. The patient was treated with thyroxine and therapeutic doses of oral steroids for hypophysitis. Similarly, Misgar et al. reported a case of infundibulo-neurohypophysitis in a 60-year-old female who presented with central diabetes insipidus and had a history of mild COVID-19 infection 8 weeks prior [8]. The patient improved

Table 8.2 Hypothalamus and pituitary dysfunction in association with SARS-CoV-2 infection and vaccination

Authors	Clinical setting	Presentation	Biochemistry	Radiology	Clinical diagnosis
Nongtait, et al. [7]	27/M Mild COVID-19 2 weeks before	Malaise, anorexia, vomiting, and early morning headache	Hyponatremia Secondary hypocortisolism, hypothyroidism, and hypogonadism Hyperprolactinemia	Diffuse enlarged pituitary, with stalk thickening and homogenous post-contrast enhancement	Lymphocytic hypophysitis
Misgar, et al. [8]	60/F Mild COVID-19 3 weeks before	Acute-onset polyuria, nocturia, and polydipsia	Hypernatremia High serum and low urine osmolality, consistent with DI The rest pituitary hormones normal	Thickened pituitary stalk with post-contrast enhancement, absent posterior pituitary bright spot	Infundibulo-neurohypophysitis
Murvelashvili, et al. [9]	51/M Second dose of SARS-CoV-2 mRNA vaccine (Moderna) 2 days before	Nausea, vomiting, and abdominal pain	Hyponatremia, secondary hypocortisolism, hypothyroidism, and hypogonadism	Homogenous enlargement of pituitary with stalk thickening Empty sella at 1-month follow-up	Acute hypophysitis
Sheikh, et al. [10]	28/M Mild COVID-19 4 weeks before	Admitted with post-viral myocarditis Developed acute-onset polyuria, nocturia, and polydipsia during course of admission	Hypernatremia Low urine osmolality with significant increase after desmopressin challenge	Normal pituitary MRI	Isolated central DI
Chua, et al. [11]	47/M Mild COVID-19 1 week before	New-onset persistent dyspepsia and eosinophilia	Low cortisol and ACTH	Normal pituitary MRI	Delayed-onset central hypocortisolism

(continued)

Table 8.2 (continued)

Authors	Clinical setting	Presentation	Biochemistry	Radiology	Clinical diagnosis
Ghosh, et al. [12]	44/F Concurrent COVID-19	Headache, projectile vomiting, visual blurring, and field defects	Hyponatremia Secondary hypocortisolism Secondary hypothyroidism on follow-up	Pituitary macroadenoma with hemorrhage	Pituitary apoplexy
Chan, et al. [13]	28/F Pregnant Concurrent COVID-19	Headache, blurring of vision, left dilated pupil, left ear pain	Secondary hypothyroidism	Pituitary macroadenoma with hemorrhage	Pituitary apoplexy
LaRoy, et al. [14]	35/M Concurrent COVID-19	Sharp, retro-orbital headache and neck stiffness	Normal hormonal evaluation	Pituitary microadenoma with hemorrhage	Pituitary apoplexy
Liew, et al. [15]	75/M Mild–moderate COVID-19 4 weeks before	Headache, fever, drowsiness, and constipation	Hyponatremia Secondary hypocortisolism, hypothyroidism, and hypogonadism	Pituitary macroadenoma with hemorrhage	Pituitary apoplexy

Abbreviations: *COVID-19* coronavirus disease 2019; *DI* diabetes insipidus; *F* female; *M* male symptomatically with oral desmopressin. Murvelashvili et al. reported a case of acute hypophysitis in a 51-year-old male who presented with nausea, vomiting, and abdominal pain 2 days following exposure to the second dose of SARS-CoV-2 mRNA vaccine (Moderna mRNA-1273 vaccine) [9]. The patient was treated with thyroxine and high dose oral steroids, to which he responded symptomatically, and a repeat imaging 1 month later revealed partial empty sella.

Isolated pituitary hormone deficiencies, namely, central diabetes insipidus and central hypocortisolism with normal pituitary imaging, have also been reported following SARS-CoV-2 infection [10, 11]. Such cases need ongoing hormone replacement and a close surveillance for any evolving pituitary deficits. Finally, cases of pituitary apoplexy, an acute medical emergency caused by hemorrhage and infarction within a pituitary adenoma, often macroadenoma, have been reported both during active infection and after recovery from acute illness [12–15]. The usual clinical presentation is headaches, vomiting, drowsiness, blurring of vision, visual field defects, cranial nerve palsies, and pituitary hormone deficits. Most patients can be managed conservatively; however, those with deteriorating level of consciousness and visual deficits need urgent neurosurgical intervention [16].

8.3 Thyroid Involvement

A variety of thyroid abnormalities have been described in the context of SARS-CoV-2 infection (Table 8.3). Like any other acute illness, low free triiodothyronine (T3), thyroxine (T4) and thyroid-stimulating hormone (TSH) levels, in line with non-thyroidal illness (NTI) syndrome, have been reported in patients admitted with COVID-19 [17, 18]. As expected, these changes resolve spontaneously in disease survivors [18]. In the THYRCOV study, Lania et al. reported a high prevalence of thyrotoxicosis (20.2%) among 287 patients hospitalized for COVID-19 in non-intensive care units [19]. The presence of thyrotoxicosis was significantly associated with higher IL-6 levels. Thyrotoxicosis was mild in most cases and resolved spontaneously during follow-up, which led authors to propose "destructive thyroiditis" as the causative mechanism.

A prospective evaluation of thyroid function at ≥3 months following the index infection was performed in 68 subjects by Clarke et al. [20], and the authors reported normal thyroid function in all study participants. They concluded that (a) thyroid function is preserved in COVID-19 survivors and (b) the symptoms of fatigue commonly seen in the post acute phase are not explained by thyroid dysfunction. Similarly, in a prospective cohort study (n=240), we reported that predominant mild and asymptomatic infection is not associated with progression of thyroid dysfunction or autoimmunity at a short-term follow-up (<1 year) [21]

There are isolated reports of subacute thyroiditis (SAT) following SARS-CoV-2 infection. SAT, also known as de Quervain thyroiditis, refers to a self-limiting inflammation of the thyroid gland that commonly ensues following a viral upper respiratory tract infection. This condition manifests as acute-onset neck pain, often radiating to the jaw, associated with fever and thyrotoxicosis symptoms. An

Table 8.3 Thyroid dysfunction in association with SARS-CoV-2 infection and vaccination

Authors	Details	Results	Conclusions
Khoo, et al. [18]	Observational cohort study. TFTs performed before, during, and after COVID-19	TSH and free T4 reduced at COVID-19 admission, compared to baseline, but spontaneously recovered on follow-up	TFT picture of non-thyroidal illness is seen in COVID-19. Thyroid function normalizes in survivors
Clarke, et al. [20]	Prospective observational study. 68 patients ≥18 years of age without baseline thyroid disease evaluated at ≥3 months following COVID-19	Normal thyroid function in all patients. Levels of thyroid hormones did not differ in patients with and without fatigue symptoms	Preserved thyroid function in COVID-19 survivors. Post-COVID-19 fatigue symptoms are not explained by thyroid dysfunction
Brancatella, et al. [24] Khatri, et al. [25]	18/F Mild COVID-19 2 weeks before 41/F Mild COVID-19 4 weeks before	Both patients presented with neck pain, fever, and thyrotoxicosis symptoms, had enlarged, tender thyroid gland on examination; diagnosed as subacute thyroiditis and successfully treated with oral steroids (cases 1 and 2) and NSAIDs (case 2)	Like other viral infections, SARS-CoV-2 can trigger subacute thyroiditis
İremli, et al. [27]	Three female healthcare workers (34–37 years) First/second dose of inactivated whole-virion SARS-CoV-2 vaccine (CoronaVac) 4–7 days before	Subacute thyroiditis, successfully managed with oral steroids in two and no treatment in one case	Subacute thyroiditis may occur following SARS-CoV-2 vaccination. Similar cases have been reported following other inactivated whole-virion (Covaxin), viral vector (Covishield), and mRNA (Moderna and Pfizer-BioNTech) vaccines [28–31]
Harris, et al. [32] Montebello, et al. [33]	18/F Mild COVID-19 16 days before 22/F Mild COVID-19 8 weeks before	Clinical and biochemical thyrotoxicosis and elevated TSH-R antibody in both cases. History of previous Graves' disease treatment in case 2	New-onset and recurrent Graves' disease can develop following SARS-CoV-2 infection

Table 8.3 (continued)

Authors	Details	Results	Conclusions
Sriphrapradang, et al. [34]	70/M Second dose of viral vector-based SARS-CoV-2 vaccine (Covishield) 2 days before	Clinical and biochemical thyrotoxicosis and elevated TSH-R antibody	Graves' disease can develop following SARS-CoV-2 vaccination. Similar cases have been reported following other SARS-CoV-2 vaccines [35, 36]

Abbreviations: *COVID-19* coronavirus disease 2019; *F* female; *M* male; *SARS-CoV-2* severe acute respiratory syndrome coronavirus 2; *T4* thyroxine; *TFT* thyroid function test; *TSH* thyroid-stimulating hormone; *TSH-R* thyroid-stimulating hormone receptor

enlarged, often asymmetric, and tender thyroid gland may be noted on physical examination. Previously, influenza, mumps, adenovirus, cytomegalovirus (CMV), rubella, and Epstein-Barr virus (EBV) have been linked to SAT [22]. SARS-CoV-2 is a new addition to this list. SAT is associated with HLA-B35, and familial occurrence and recurrent episodes are linked to this high-risk genotype [23]. Thus, SAT occurs through susceptibility to viral infection in genetically predisposed individuals. SAT often runs a triphasic course, characterized by thyrotoxicosis with decreased radioactive iodine uptake, followed by hypothyroidism and, eventually, euthyroidism.

Nearly 90% of patients show complete and spontaneous recovery of thyroid function; the remaining 10% develop permanent hypothyroidism and need long-term replacement. Treatment is mainly symptomatic and comprises beta-blockers for thyrotoxicosis symptoms and nonsteroidal anti-inflammatory drugs (NSAIDs) for neck pain. A trial of oral steroids is indicated for patients with severe neck pain or no response to NSAIDs. A suggested regimen is oral prednisolone 15–25 mg/day for 2 weeks, followed by taper over the next 4–6 weeks. The first case of SAT following SARS-CoV-2 was reported by Brancatella et al. in an 18-year-old female [24]. She presented 2 weeks following the infection with typical symptoms and was successfully treated with a course of oral steroids. Similarly, Khatri et al. reported post-SARS-CoV-2 SAT in a 41-year-old male who was treated successfully with oral NSAIDs [25]. Thyroid function outcomes in patients admitted with SARS-CoV-2-associated thyrotoxicosis, related to subacute thyroiditis, were reported in a study by Pizzocaro et al. [26]. At a median follow-up of 90 days, thyroid function spontaneously normalized in most (28, 97%) patients, and only 1 developed hypothyroidism

Similar to influenza, H1N1, and hepatitis B vaccines, different SARS-CoV-2 vaccines have been reported to trigger SAT. Cases have been reported following exposure to inactivated whole-virion (e.g., CoronaVac (Sinovac Life Sciences) and Covaxin (BBV152)), viral vector (e.g., Covishield (ChAdOx1 nCoV-19)), and mRNA (e.g., Moderna mRNA-1273 and Pfizer-BioNTech (BNT162b2)) vaccines [27–31]. In this scenario, SAT reflects postvaccination autoimmune/inflammatory syndrome induced by adjuvants (ASIA) that occurs following exposure to vaccine adjuvants in genetically predisposed individuals [27]. Notably, adjuvants (such as aluminum hydroxide) are used to enhance the immunogenicity of viral antigen and induce a better adaptive immune syndrome. Postvaccination ASIA is a well-described entity, and other endocrinopathies previously reported under this syndrome include type 1 diabetes, premature ovarian failure, autoimmune thyroid disease, and adrenal insufficiency [27].

SARS-CoV-2 infection and vaccination are also known to trigger Graves' disease [32–36], an autoimmune form of hyperthyroidism characterized by the presence of stimulatory antibodies against TSH receptors. Clinically, this condition manifests as goiter, hyperthyroidism, and, in some cases, infiltrative orbitopathy and dermopathy. Graves' disease is postulated to occur following exposure to environmental agents in genetically predisposed individuals. The known environmental triggers include viral infection (e.g., Coxsackie B virus), drugs (e.g., alemtuzumab, ipilimumab), iodine, smoking, and stress. SARS-CoV-2 infection is a new addition to this list of environmental triggers. The proposed mechanisms include (a) triggering of the immunological cascade by the severe pro-inflammatory state of infection, (b) molecular mimicry, and (c) infection-related stress [32]. Subacute thyroiditis is an important differential diagnosis of this condition. Prolonged duration of symptoms, the presence of a prominent goiter, orbitopathy/dermopathy, features of other autoimmune disease such as vitiligo, a high T3/T4 ratio, and diffusely increased thyroidal radioactive iodine uptake all favor the diagnosis of Graves' disease. Notably, the recent use of iodinated contrast agent (within the preceding 3 months) may saturate thyroidal iodine pool and impair radioiodine uptake. A TSH-receptor antibody test may be helpful in such cases, as in pregnancy, where radioactive iodine scan is contraindicated. Management options include antithyroid drugs, radioactive iodine ablation, and thyroidectomy; the reader is directed to an excellent review for more details [37].

8.4 Endocrine Pancreatic Abnormalities

It is well known that diabetes is associated with poor COVID-19 outcomes [38]. Recent data also suggest increased susceptibility to SARS-CoV-2 infection among persons with diabetes [39, 40]. Furthermore, SARS-CoV-2 may itself induce metabolic dysfunction and new-onset diabetes (Table 8.4) [41–43]. In this regard, a global registry of COVID-19-related diabetes has been established [44]. This registry defines new-onset diabetes following COVID-19 as follows: (a) confirmed SARS-CoV-2 infection, (b) no past history of diabetes, and (c) a previously normal glycated hemoglobin (HbA1c) level. The precise mechanisms are unknown, but multiple factors may contribute, including pre-existing undiagnosed diabetes, stress-related hyperglycemia, steroid-induced hyperglycemia, and the direct/indirect effects of SARS-CoV-2 on the pancreatic beta cell [41].

Table 8.4 New-onset diabetes (NOD) in association with SARS-CoV-2 infection

Authors	Details	Results	Conclusions
Huang, et al. [42]	Ambidirectional cohort study 1733 patients admitted for COVID-19 evaluated at a median follow-up of 6 months	New-onset diabetes in 3.3% of patients	Extrapulmonary manifestations, including diabetes may appear as a part of post-COVID-19 syndrome
Ayoubkhani, et al. [43]	Retrospective cohort study 47,780 patients admitted for COVID-19 evaluated at a mean follow-up of 140 days	New-onset diabetes in 4.9% of patients	Same as above
Ghosh, et al. [48]	Retrospective cohort study 282 patients with NOD before COVID-19 pandemic (September 2019–February 2020) compared with 273 patients with NOD during the pandemic (April–October 2020)	Patients with NOD during the pandemic had higher fasting and postprandial blood glucose and glycated hemoglobin, compared to those diagnosed before the pandemic No difference in C-peptide or glycemic parameters in patients with NOD during the pandemic who tested positive or negative for COVID-19 antibody	Individuals with NOD during the pandemic had more severe glycemic parameters at diagnosis; however, they did not differ in symptomatology and phenotype
Goyal, et al. [56]	Prospective cohort study 352 participants, without baseline diabetes, evaluated at two time points: pre-COVID-19 (2016–2019) and peri-COVID-19 (2020–2021). SARS-CoV-2 antibody test at the second visit to determine infection Glycemic progression between visits defined as conversion from normoglycemia to prediabetes/diabetes and from prediabetes to diabetes	159 (45.2%) participants in the cohort had SARS-CoV-2 infection. Of these, 122 (76.7%) had mild/asymptomatic infection Progression in glycemic category not significantly different between the infected and noninfected groups. Similarly, the two groups were not different in terms of progression of insulin indices (HOMA-IR, oDI, Matsuda index)	Predominant mild/asymptomatic SARS-CoV-2 infection was not associated with glycemic progression or worsening of beta cell function and insulin resistance

Abbreviations: *COVID-19* coronavirus disease 2019; *HOMA-IR* homeostasis model assessment of insulin resistance; *NOD* new-onset diabetes; *oDI* oral disposition index; *SARS-CoV-2* severe acute respiratory syndrome coronavirus 2

In a multicenter study from London, Unsworth et al. reported an 80% increase in new-onset type 1 diabetes during the pandemic, compared with previous years [45]. To the contrary, a study by Tittel et al., which pooled data from 216 pediatric centers in Germany, reported no such increase [46]. Notably, both the cohorts demonstrated an increased severity of diabetes at presentation, with significant increases in the proportion of diabetic ketoacidosis (DKA) and severe DKA at the time of diagnosis [45, 47]. The reasons could be multiple and include (a) delayed presentation due to fear of contracting virus and reduced medical care for non-COVID-19 illnesses, (b) complex psychosocial factors, and (c) SARS-CoV-2-related insulinopenia and rise in pro-inflammatory cytokines. Similarly, a retrospective study by Ghosh et al. found that patients with new-onset diabetes diagnosed during the pandemic had higher fasting and postprandial blood glucose and glycated hemoglobin levels than those diagnosed before the pandemic [48]. However, there was no difference in C-peptide levels or glycemic parameters between seropositive and seronegative patients diagnosed during the pandemic. Recently, there have been reports of hyperglycemic emergencies [DKA and hyperglycemic hyperosmolar state (HHS)] following COVID-19 vaccination in patients with poorly controlled type 1 and type 2 diabetes [49–53]. These events occurred within 1–6 weeks following the exposure to various SARS-CoV-2 vaccines, including inactivated whole-virion (Covaxin (BBV152)), viral vector (Covishield (ChAdOx1 nCoV-19)), and mRNA (e.g., Moderna mRNA-1273 and Pfizer-BioNTech (BNT162b2)) vaccines. It is therefore advisable that patients with diabetes, especially those with suboptimal glycemic control, be closely monitored for hyperglycemia and ketosis in the initial few weeks following the vaccination [49].

Various autopsy studies have confirmed that SARS-CoV-2 infects beta cells and leads to beta cell apoptosis, loss of insulin secretion, and transdifferentiation into glucagon-producing alpha cells [54, 55]. However, most data on new-onset diabetes have been derived from hospitalized patients, who often suffer from more severe disease than those in the community. To address this lacuna, we performed a longitudinal study, wherein 352 healthy participants from an established cohort were evaluated in pre-COVID-19 (2016–2019) and peri-COVID-19 (2020–2021) periods for progression of glycemic and cardiometabolic variables [56]. The study was performed before the onset of the national vaccination program, and therefore, seropositivity (for SARS-CoV-2 IgG) was a surrogate for viral infection. A total of 159 (45.2%) participants had SARS-CoV-2 infection, of whom 122 (76.7%) had mild/asymptomatic infection, representative of the real-world scenario. The progression of glycemic categories, i.e., from normal glucose tolerance to prediabetes or diabetes and from prediabetes to diabetes, was not significantly different between infected (20.8%) and noninfected (19.7%) groups. Thus, we concluded that predominant mild/asymptomatic infection is not associated with worsening of glycemic parameters and excessive development of new-onset diabetes, at least on a short-term follow-up. More prospective studies are needed globally, involving different patient populations and at a longer duration following the index infection to delineate the burden and pathophysiology of SARS-CoV-2-induced new-onset diabetes. Such data should also clarify whether new-onset diabetes is a permanent condition or not.

Until such time, clinicians should watch for metabolic dysfunction in patients with a history of SARS-CoV-2 infection.

8.5 Adrenal Involvement

Glucocorticoids have been widely used in COVID-19 for their anti-inflammatory properties, especially in patients with the moderate-severe disease. In the post-acute phase, there is always a risk for secondary adrenal insufficiency following abrupt withdrawal or even exogenous Cushing's syndrome following unsupervised prolonged use of glucocorticoids [57, 58]. The risk increases with the use of more potent and long-acting formulations (e.g., dexamethasone, methylprednisolone, and prednisolone in that order), a higher dose (e.g., prednisolone 40 mg/day equivalent or more), a longer treatment duration (e.g., more than 7–14 days), and administration at a nonphysiological time of the day (e.g., evening-night, compared to morning-afternoon hours) [57]. Primary adrenal dysfunction has been reported less often in the context of COVID-19 (Table 8.5). In a prospective evaluation of the

Table 8.5 Adrenal dysfunction in association with SARS-CoV-2 infection and vaccination

Authors	Details	Results	Conclusions
Clarke, et al. [20]	Prospective observational study. 70 patients ≥18 years of age evaluated at ≥3 months following COVID-19	All patients had peak cortisol ≥450 nmol/L after Synacthen stimulation. Levels of basal and peak cortisol did not differ in patients with and without fatigue symptoms	Preserved adrenal function in COVID-19 survivors. Post-COVID-19 fatigue symptoms are not explained by adrenal dysfunction
Frankel, et al. [59]	66/F Concurrent COVID-19 Known case of APLA syndrome	Primary adrenal insufficiency due to bilateral adrenal hemorrhage. Persistent glucocorticoid and mineralocorticoid requirement 4 weeks after recovery from infection	Like other infections, SARS-CoV-2 can precipitate adrenal hemorrhage and result in primary adrenal insufficiency
Taylor, et al. [60]	38/M First dose of adenoviral vector SARS-CoV-2 vaccine (Covishield) 8 days before	Bilateral adrenal hemorrhage and primary adrenal insufficiency. Diagnosed as VITT and managed accordingly	VITT is a rare complication of adenoviral vector-based vaccines that may manifest as adrenal hemorrhage
Sanchez, et al. [61]	64/F Mild COVID-19 5 months before	Clinical and biochemical features of primary adrenal insufficiency. Positive anti-21 hydroxylase antibodies	SARS-CoV-2 can promote the development or progression of autoimmune adrenal insufficiency

Abbreviations: *COVID-19* coronavirus disease 2019; *F* female; *M* male; *SARS-CoV-2* severe acute respiratory syndrome coronavirus 2; *VITT* vaccine-induced thrombosis and thrombocytopenia adrenal function at ≥3 months following the index infection, Clarke et al. reported a peak post-Synacthen (ACTH 1–24) cortisol level ≥ 450 nmol/L (18 μg/dL) in all study participants (n = 70), suggestive of preserved adrenal function [20]. Moreover, baseline or peak cortisol levels were not different in patients with and without fatigue, confirming that adrenal dysfunction does not explain post-COVID-19 fatigue symptoms.

Isolated case reports indicate that SARS-CoV-2 may lead to the progression or development of primary adrenal insufficiency through adrenal hemorrhage or by inducing autoimmunity. Adrenal hemorrhage presents with nonspecific signs and symptoms, including abdominal pain and tenderness, nausea, vomiting, fatigue, fever, and hypotension. Pathogenesis involves increased arterial inflow during a stressful event coupled with reduced venous drainage, resulting in vascular congestion and hemorrhage. Frankel et al. reported a case of acute COVID-19 associated with primary adrenal insufficiency and bilateral adrenal hemorrhage in a 66-year-old female with a background history of APLA syndrome [59]. The patient recovered completely from acute illness but had persistent glucocorticoid and mineralocorticoid requirements at 4 weeks. Similarly, Taylor et al. reported a case of bilateral adrenal hemorrhage and adrenal insufficiency in a 38-year-old male, 8 days after receiving the first dose of adenoviral vector-based SARS-CoV-2 vaccine (Covishield (ChAdOx1 nCoV-19)) [60]. This adverse event represented a manifestation of vaccine-induced thrombosis and thrombocytopenia (VITT), a prothrombotic syndrome with thrombocytopenia rarely reported in subjects receiving adenoviral vector-based vaccines. Finally, Sanchez et al. reported autoimmune adrenal insufficiency in a 64-year-old female, possibly related to mild COVID-19 she had 5 months prior [61]. Thus, although rare, clinicians should consider primary adrenal insufficiency as a differential diagnosis in patients who present with suggestive symptoms during or after the acute illness.

8.6 Gonadal Involvement

SARS-CoV-2 entry receptor, ACE2, is highly expressed in human testicular tissue, including spermatogonia, Leydig cells, and Sertoli cells [62]. Orchitis and germ cell damage were reported in the previous SARS outbreak [63]. In hospitalized patients with COVID-19, a pattern of elevated luteinizing hormone (LH) and maintained testosterone have been reported, suggestive of an early testicular dysfunction [64]. Postmortem examination of 12 patients who died of COVID-19 revealed a significant seminiferous tubular injury, reduced Leydig cells, and interstitial inflammation [65]. However, the SARS-CoV-2 was not detected in the testis by polymerase chain reaction (PCR) in a majority (90%) of subjects. The mechanisms for testicular dysfunction include direct damage by the virus and inflammatory/immunological orchitis [66].

A recent study by Moreno-Perez et al. evaluated Leydig and Sertoli cell dysfunction in a cohort of 143 males with a median age of 59 years, enrolled at 8–12 weeks

Table 8.6 Gonadal dysfunction in association with SARS-CoV-2 infection

Authors	Details	Results	Conclusions
Moreno-Perez, et al. [67]	Cross-sectional study 144 patients evaluated 8–12 weeks after recovery from COVID-19. Of these, 72% had severe pneumonia Low testosterone defined as total testosterone level < 2 ng/ml or level 2–4 ng/ml with free testosterone <6.34 ng/dl. Sertoli cell dysfunction defined as inhibin B < 89 pg/ml	Low testosterone in 41 (28.7%) and Sertoli cell dysfunction in 25 (18.1%) participants. Obesity and hypokalemia were predictors of low testosterone, while age > 65 years predicted Sertoli cell dysfunction	High prevalence of low testosterone and Sertoli cell dysfunction in severe COVID-19 survivors

Abbreviations: *COVID-19* coronavirus disease 2019

following recovery from COVID-19 (Table 8.6) [67]. A majority of participants (72%) had a history of severe pneumonia. "Low testosterone," defined as total testosterone <200 ng/dL or calculated free testosterone <6.36 ng/dL in those with total testosterone of 200–400 ng/dL, was found in 41 (28.7%) participants. Among these, 22% had high LH levels, suggestive of primary testicular dysfunction, while 78% had low or inappropriately normal LH, suggestive of impairment of hypothalamic-pituitary-gonadal axis. Sertoli cell dysfunction, defined as serum inhibin <89 pg/ml, was found in 25 (18.1%) participants. The presence of obesity and hypokalemia predicted "low testosterone," while age >65 years was predictive of Sertoli cell dysfunction. This study highlights a relatively high prevalence of male hypogonadism in COVID-19 survivors. However, the study was limited by (a) short follow-up duration, and therefore, it remains to be seen whether these changes are transient or permanent, (b) inclusion of a relatively older population with higher disease severity at baseline, (c) pre-existing hypogonadism that was not excluded since pre-COVID-19 hormonal levels were not available, (d) semen analysis that was not performed, and (e) testosterone measurement that was not repeated and performed using a non-mass spectrometric method. While prospective studies that address these limitations are needed in the future, clinicians should maintain a close vigil and consider COVID-19-induced testicular dysfunction in an appropriate clinical scenario.

Data on SARS-CoV-2 infection and female gonadal and reproductive function are limited. In their experiments, Goad et al. demonstrated that SARS-CoV-2 receptors, ACE2, and TMPRSS2 are not expressed at significant levels in the female reproductive tract [68]. Accordingly, it is expected that the viral infection does not have a major impact on this organ system [69]. In a retrospective study, Li et al. described transient menstrual changes, mainly decreased flow and increased intermenstrual interval, in 177 COVID-19 patients of childbearing age [70]. Notably, menstrual cycles returned to normal within 1–2 months following discharge in 99%

of cases. Furthermore, the mean sex hormone and AMH concentrations in such patients were similar to those of age-matched controls.

8.7 Take-Home Message

- Endocrine abnormalities reported following COVID-19 include hypophysitis, isolated pituitary hormone deficiency and apoplexy (hypothalamus and pituitary), subacute thyroiditis and Graves' disease (thyroid), new-onset diabetes (pancreas), adrenal hemorrhage and primary adrenal insufficiency (adrenals), and male hypogonadism (testis).
- Post-COVID-19 endocrinopathies often manifest within 3–6 months following the index infection and result either from direct damage by the virus or indirect inflammatory/immunological damage.
- Endocrine adverse events have also been reported following different SARS-CoV-2 vaccines, including inactivated whole-virion, viral vector-based, and mRNA vaccines.
- Vaccine-induced endocrinopathies are extremely rare and should not discourage the general public from being vaccinated since the benefits of vaccination far outweigh the small potential risks.
- Clinicians caring for patients with COVID-19 should suspect endocrine complications in appropriate clinical scenarios and report any new and previously unknown manifestations.

Conflicts of Interest None

Funding None

References

1. Beyerstedt S, Casaro EB, Rangel ÉB. COVID-19: angiotensin-converting enzyme 2 (ACE2) expression and tissue susceptibility to SARS-CoV-2 infection. Eur J Clin Microbiol Infect Dis. 2021;40(5):905–19.
2. Somasundaram NP, Ranathunga I, Ratnasamy V, Wijewickrama PSA, Dissanayake HA, Yogendranathan N, et al. The impact of SARS-Cov-2 virus infection on the endocrine system. J Endocr Soc. 2020;4(8):bvaa082.
3. Ehrenfeld M, Tincani A, Andreoli L, Cattalini M, Greenbaum A, Kanduc D, et al. Covid-19 and autoimmunity. Autoimmun Rev. 2020;19(8):102597.
4. Leow MK, Kwek DS, Ng AW, Ong KC, Kaw GJ, Lee LS. Hypocortisolism in survivors of severe acute respiratory syndrome (SARS). Clin Endocrinol. 2005;63(2):197–202.
5. Wheatland R. Molecular mimicry of ACTH in SARS–implications for corticosteroid treatment and prophylaxis. Med Hypotheses. 2004;63(5):855–62.

6. Frara S, Allora A, Castellino L, di Filippo L, Loli P, Giustina A. COVID-19 and the pituitary. Pituitary. 2021;24(3):465–81.
7. Nonglait PL, Naik R, Raizada N. Hypophysitis after COVID-19 infection. Indian J Endocrinol Metab. 2021;25(3):255–6.
8. Misgar RA, Rasool A, Wani AI, Bashir MI. Central diabetes insipidus (Infundibuloneurohypophysitis): a late complication of COVID-19 infection. J Endocrinol Investig. 2021;44(12):2855–6.
9. Murvelashvili N, Tessnow A. A case of Hypophysitis following immunization with the mRNA-1273 SARS-CoV-2 vaccine. J Investig Med High Impact Case Rep. 2021c;9:23247096211043386.
10. Sheikh AB, Javed N, Sheikh AAE, Upadhyay S, Shekhar R. Diabetes insipidus and concomitant myocarditis: a late sequelae of COVID-19 infection. J Investig Med High Impact Case Rep. 2021;9:2324709621999954.
11. Chua MWJ, Chua MPW. Delayed onset of central Hypocortisolism in a patient recovering from COVID-19. AACE Clin Case Rep. 2021;7(1):2–5.
12. Ghosh R, Roy D, Roy D, Mandal A, Dutta A, Naga D, et al. A rare case of SARS-CoV-2 infection associated with pituitary apoplexy without comorbidities. J Endocr Soc. 2021;5(3):bvaa203.
13. Chan JL, Gregory KD, Smithson SS, Naqvi M, Mamelak AN. Pituitary apoplexy associated with acute COVID-19 infection and pregnancy. Pituitary. 2020;23(6):716–20.
14. LaRoy M, McGuire M. Pituitary apoplexy in the setting of COVID-19 infection. Am J Emerg Med. 2021;47:329.e1–2.
15. Liew SY, Seese R, Shames A, Majumdar K. Apoplexy in a previously undiagnosed pituitary macroadenoma in the setting of recent COVID-19 infection. BMJ Case Rep. 2021;14(7):e243607.
16. Ranabir S, Baruah MP. Pituitary apoplexy. Indian. J Endocrinol Metab. 2011;15(Suppl 3):S188 96.
17. Kumar B, Gopalakrishnan M, Garg MK, Purohit P, Banerjee M, Sharma P, et al. Endocrine dysfunction among patients with COVID-19: a single-Centre experience from a tertiary hospital in India. Indian J Endocr Metab. 2021;25:14–9.
18. Khoo B, Tan T, Clarke SA, Mills EG, Patel B, Modi M, et al. Thyroid function before, during, and after COVID-19. J Clin Endocrinol Metab. 2021;106(2):e803–11.
19. Lania A, Sandri MT, Cellini M, Mirani M, Lavezzi E, Mazziotti G. Thyrotoxicosis in patients with COVID-19: the THYRCOV study. Eur J Endocrinol. 2020;183:381–7.
20. Clarke SA, Phylactou M, Patel B, Mills EG, Muzi B, Izzi-Engbeaya C, et al. Normal adrenal and thyroid function in patients who survive COVID-19 infection. J Clin Endocrinol Metab. 2021;106(8):2208–20.
21. Goyal A, Gupta Y, Kalaivani M, Tandon N. Mild and asymptomatic SARS-CoV-2 infection is not associated with progression of thyroid dysfunction or thyroid autoimmunity. Clin Endocrinol (Oxf). 2022 Apr 5:. https://doi.org/10.1111/cen.14731.
22. Desailloud R, Hober D. Viruses and thyroiditis: an update. Virol J. 2009;6:5.
23. Nyulassy S, Hnilica P, Buc M, Guman M, Hirschova V, Stefanovic J. Subacute (de Quervain's) thyroiditis: association with HLA-Bw35 antigen and abnormalities of the complement system, immunoglobulins and other serum proteins. J Clin Endocrinol Metab. 1977;45:270–4.
24. Brancatella A, Ricci D, Viola N, Sgrò D, Santini F, Latrofa F. Subacute thyroiditis after Sars-COV-2 infection. J Clin Endocrinol Metab. 2020;105(7):dgaa276.
25. Khatri A, Charlap E, Kim A. Subacute thyroiditis from COVID-19 infection: a case report and review of literature. Eur Thyroid J. 2021;9(6):324–8.
26. Pizzocaro A, Colombo P, Vena W, Ariano S, Magnoni P, Reggiani F, et al. Outcome of Sars-COV-2-related thyrotoxicosis in survivors of Covid-19: a prospective study. Endocrine. 2021;73(2):255–60.
27. İremli BG, Şendur SN, Ünlütürk U. Three cases of subacute thyroiditis following SARS-CoV-2 vaccine: Postvaccination ASIA syndrome. J Clin Endocrinol Metab. 2021;106(9):2600–5.
28. Soltanpoor P, Norouzi G. Subacute thyroiditis following COVID-19 vaccination. Clin Case Rep. 2021;9(10):e04812.

29. Oyibo SO. Subacute thyroiditis after receiving the adenovirus-vectored vaccine for coronavirus disease (COVID-19). Cureus. 2021;13(6):e16045.
30. Plaza-Enriquez L, Khatiwada P, Sanchez-Valenzuela M, Sikha A. A case report of subacute thyroiditis following mRNA COVID-19 vaccine. Case Rep Endocrinol. 2021;2021:8952048.
31. Sözen M, Topaloğlu Ö, Çetinarslan B, Selek A, Cantürk Z, Gezer E, et al. COVID-19 mRNA vaccine may trigger subacute thyroiditis. Hum VaccinImmunother. 2021:1–6.
32. Harris A, Al MM. Graves' thyrotoxicosis following SARS-CoV-2 infection. AACE Clin Case Rep. 2021;7(1):14–6.
33. Montebello A. Recurrent Graves' disease post SARS-CoV-2 infection. BMJ Case Rep. 2021;14(8):e244714.
34. Sriphrapradang C, Shantavasinkul PC. Graves' disease following SARS-CoV-2 vaccination. Endocrine. 2021;74(3):473–4.
35. Lui DTW, Lee KK, Lee CH, Lee ACH, Hung IFN, Tan KCB. Development of Graves' disease after SARS-CoV-2 mRNA vaccination: a case report and literature review. Front Public Health. 2021;9:778964.
36. Vera-Lastra O, Ordinola Navarro A, Cruz Domiguez MP, Medina G, Sánchez Valadez TI, Jara LJ. Two cases of Graves' disease following SARS-CoV-2 vaccination: an autoimmune/inflammatory syndrome induced by adjuvants. Thyroid. 2021;31(9):1436–9.
37. Smith TJ, Hegedüs L. Graves' disease. N Engl J Med. 2016;375(16):1552–65.
38. de Almeida-Pititto B, Dualib PM, Zajdenverg L, et al. Severity and mortality of COVID 19 in patients with diabetes, hypertension and cardiovascular disease: a meta-analysis. Diabetol Metab Syndr. 2020;12:75.
39. Goyal A, Gupta Y, Kalaivani M, Praveen PA, Ambekar S, Tandon N. SARS-CoV-2 Seroprevalence in individuals with type 1 and type 2 diabetes compared with controls. Endocr Pract. 2021;S1530-891X(21):01416.
40. Yadav R, Acharjee A, Salkar A, et al. Mumbai mayhem of COVID-19 pandemic reveals important factors that influence susceptibility to infection. E Clin Med. 2021;35:100841.
41. Khunti K, Del Prato S, Mathieu C, Kahn SE, Gabbay RA, Buse JB. COVID-19, hyperglycemia, and new-onset diabetes. Diabetes Care. 2021;44(12):2645–55.
42. Huang C, Huang L, Wang Y, et al. 6-month consequences of COVID-19 in patients discharged from hospital: a cohort study. Lancet. 2021;397:220–32.
43. Ayoubkhani D, Khunti K, Nafilyan V, et al. Post-covid syndrome in individuals admitted to hospital with COVID-19: retrospective cohort study. BMJ. 2021;372:n693.
44. Rubino F, Amiel SA, Zimmet P, et al. New-onset diabetes in Covid-19. N Engl J Med. 2020;383(8):789–90.
45. Unsworth R, Wallace S, Oliver NS, et al. New-onset type 1 diabetes in children during COVID-19: multicenter regional findings in the U.K. Diabetes Care. 2020;43:e170–1.
46. Tittel SR, Rosenbauer J, Kamrath C, et al. DPV initiative. Did the COVID-19 lockdown affect the incidence of pediatric type 1 diabetes in Germany? Diabetes Care. 2020;43:e172–3.
47. Kamrath C, Mönkemöller K, Biester T, et al. Ketoacidosis in children and adolescents with newly diagnosed type 1 diabetes during the COVID-19 pandemic in Germany. JAMA. 2020;324:801–4.
48. Ghosh A, Anjana RM, Shanthi Rani CS, et al. Glycemic parameters in patients with new-onset diabetes during COVID-19 pandemic are more severe than in patients with new-onset diabetes before the pandemic: NOD COVID India study. Diabetes Metab Syndr. 2021;15:215–22.
49. Ganakumar V, Jethwani P, Roy A, Shukla R, Mittal M, Garg MK. Diabetic ketoacidosis (DKA) in type 1 diabetes mellitus (T1DM) temporally related to COVID-19 vaccination. Diabetes Metab Syndr. 2021;16(1):102371.
50. Zilbermint M, Demidowich AP. Severe diabetic ketoacidosis after the second dose of mRNA-1273 COVID-19 vaccine. J Diabetes Sci Technol. 2022;16(1):248–9.
51. Abu-Rumaileh MA, Gharaibeh AM, Gharaibeh NE. COVID-19 vaccine and hyperosmolar hyperglycemic state. Cureus. 13(3):e14125.
52. Lee HJ, Sajan A, Tomer Y. Hyperglycemic emergencies associated with COVID-19 vaccination: a case series and discussion. J Endocr Soc. 2021 Sep 25;5(11):bvab141.

53. Edwards AE, Vathenen R, Henson SM, Finer S, Gunganah K. Acute hyperglycaemic crisis after vaccination against COVID-19: a case series. Diabet Med. 2021;38(11):e14631.
54. Wu CT, Lidsky PV, Xiao Y, et al. SARS-CoV-2 infects human pancreatic β cells and elicits β cell impairment. Cell Metab. 2021;33(8):1565–1576.e5.
55. Tang X, Uhl S, Zhang T, et al. SARS-CoV-2 infection induces beta cell transdifferentiation. Cell Metab. 2021;33(8):1577–1591.e7.
56. Goyal A, Gupta Y, Kalaivani M, Bhatla N, Tandon N. Impact of SARS-CoV-2 on progression of glycemic and Cardiometabolic variables and changes in insulin indices: a longitudinal study. Diabetes Ther. 2021;12(11):3011–23.
57. Ferraù F, Ceccato F, Cannavò S, Scaroni C. What we have to know about corticosteroids use during Sars-Cov-2 infection. J Endocrinol Investig. 2021;44(4):693–701. https://doi.org/10.1007/s40618-020-01384-5.
58. Alessi J, de Oliveira GB, Schaan BD, et al. Dexamethasone in the era of COVID-19: friend or foe? An essay on the effects of dexamethasone and the potential risks of its inadvertent use in patients with diabetes. Diabetol Metab Syndr. 2020;12:80.
59. Frankel M, Feldman I, Levine M, Frank Y, Bogot NR, Benjaminov O, Kurd R, et al. Bilateral adrenal hemorrhage in coronavirus disease 2019 patient: a case report. J Clin Endocrinol Metab. 2020;105(12):dgaa487.
60. Taylor P, Allen L, Shrikrishnapalasuriyar N, Stechman M, Rees A. Vaccine-induced thrombosis and thrombocytopenia with bilateral adrenal haemorrhage. Clin Endocrinol. 2021; https://doi.org/10.1111/cen.14548.
61. Sánchez J, Cohen M, Zapater JL, Eisenberg Y. Primary adrenal insufficiency after COVID-19 infection. AACE Clin Case Rep. 2021; https://doi.org/10.1016/j.aace.2021.11.001.
62. Wang Z, Xu X. scRNA-seq profiling of human testes reveals the presence of the ACE2 receptor, a target for SARS-CoV-2 infection in spermatogonia, Leydig and Sertoli cells. Cell. 2020;9(4):920.
63. Xu J, Qi L, Chi X, et al. Orchitis: a complication of severe acute respiratory syndrome (SARS). Biol Reprod. 2006;74(2):410–6. https://doi.org/10.1095/biolreprod.105.044776.
64. Ma Y, Pei S, Shaman J, Dubrow R, Chen K. Effect of SARS-CoV-2 infection upon male gonadal function: a single center-based study [published online ahead of print March 30, 2020]. *medRxiv*. https://doi.org/10.1101/2020.03.21.20037267.
65. Yang M, Chen S, Huang B, et al. Pathological findings in the testes of COVID-19 patients: clinical implications. Eur Urol Focus. 2020;6(5):1124–9.
66. Illiano E, Trama F, Costantini E. Could COVID-19 have an impact on male fertility? Andrologia. 2020;52(6):e13654. https://doi.org/10.1111/and.1365.
67. Moreno-Perez O, Merino E, Alfayate R, Torregrosa ME, Andres M, Leon-Ramirez JM, et al. Male pituitary-gonadal axis dysfunction in post-acute COVID-19 syndrome-prevalence and associated factors: a Mediterranean case series. Clin Endocrinol. 2021; https://doi.org/10.1111/cen.14537.
68. Goad J, Rudolph J, Rajkovic A. Female reproductive tract has low concentration of SARS-CoV2 receptors. PLoS One. 2020 Dec 14;15(12):e0243959. https://doi.org/10.1371/journal.pone.0243959.
69. Madhu SV, Raizada N. COVID-19 and endocrine disorders - emerging links in this puzzle. Ind J Endocrinol Metab. 2021;25(1):1–3. https://doi.org/10.4103/2230-8210.322027.
70. Li K, Chen G, Hou H, Liao Q, Chen J, Bai H, et al. Analysis of sex hormones and menstruation in COVID-19 women of child-bearing age. Reprod Biomed Online. 2021;42:260–7.

Renal Abnormalities Following COVID-19

9

S. Arunkumar and Sanjay Kumar Agarwal

The ongoing COVID-19 pandemic has affected millions of lives adversely in the last 2 years, and the future course of the pandemic remains unknown. Initially, COVID-19 infection was thought to be an acute respiratory illness, but slowly it became clear that it is a multi-system disease involving almost all body organs. Still more alarming is the realization that this infection is not as "acute" only as previously believed but has lasting effects in various organ systems. Kidneys are no exception, not only being involved during acute COVID-19 infection in multiple ways but also are important organs, in which infection leads to chronic kidney disease with varying manifestations. This review will restrict the majority of the discussion to long-term sequelae of COVID-19 concerning kidneys.

9.1 Understanding Basic Kidney Syndrome

Before discussing long-term kidney consequences, it will be prudent to know common kidney syndromes, which will help understand kidney abnormalities following COVID-19.

A. *Acute kidney injury*: This is defined as a recent onset of renal dysfunction manifested by an elevation of serum creatinine; therefore fall in estimated glomerular filtration rate (eGFR) with or without oliguria, and patients may recover in more than 80–90% of cases. However, approximately 10–20% of patients with severe acute kidney injury (AKI) remain at risk of developing chronic kidney disease (CKD) [1].
B. *Chronic kidney disease:* It is defined as evidence of renal disease present for >3 months with or without decrease in eGFR <60 ml/min. Evidence of a renal

S. Arunkumar · S. K. Agarwal (✉)
Department of Nephrology, AIIMS, New Delhi, India

A. Mohan, S. Mittal (eds.), *Post COVID-19 Complications and Management*,
https://doi.org/10.1007/978-981-19-4407-9_9

disease is usually in the form of abnormal urinary protein loss of >30 mg/day, urinary sediment anomalies (RBC, WBC, casts, etc.), and/or radiological renal abnormality [2]. Once correctly diagnosed, CKD does not recover and tends to progress to more advanced kidney disease, a stage called end-stage kidney disease (ESKD). At the ESKD, the patient cannot be managed with only medical treatment and will need renal replacement therapy (RRT) in the form of dialysis and/or renal transplant.

C. *Glomerular diseases*: Many renal diseases involve the glomerulus and are grouped under the heading glomerular diseases. The two most important criteria for defining glomerular diseases are significant proteinuria (> 1.0 g/day) and glomerular hematuria (dysmorphic RBCs and/or RBC casts). Based upon the degree of proteinuria, kidney dysfunction, and rapidity of onset of disease, the glomerular diseases are subdivided into clinical syndromes such as acute glomerulonephritis (AGN), nephrotic syndrome (NS), acute nephritic syndrome, rapidly progressive GN (RPGN), chronic glomerulonephritis (CGN), and asymptomatic urinary abnormalities (AUA).

D. *Hypertension*: Most (around 90%) patients of hypertension in the community are primary hypertension, but among the 10% cases of secondary hypertension, kidney diseases remain the most common cause.

9.2 Renal Diseases and COVID-19

Kidney diseases are important risk factors for acquiring COVID-19 infection because of kidney patients' immunocompromised status, which may be due to the intake of immunosuppressive drugs or the intrinsic nature of their disease condition. The following broad category of patients concerning kidney disease may get COVID-19 infection:

1. A healthy person with normal kidney functions
2. Patients with kidney diseases on immunosuppression
   - Kidney disease patients on immunosuppressive medication
   - Kidney transplant patients
3. Patients with pre-existing CKD
   - CKD of varying severity and varying etiology
   - Kidney transplant patients with graft dysfunction
4. Patients on dialysis: peritoneal dialysis or hemodialysis

9.3 Acute COVID-19 and Kidney Involvement

Kidney involvement in COVID-19 can range from asymptomatic urinary abnormalities, including varying degrees of proteinuria and hematuria, to kidney dysfunction presenting as AKI, which may require RRT in selected cases. AKI affects around 20–40% of critically ill COVID-19 patients. Renal replacement therapy during hospitalization is required in 5–10% of all COVID-19 patients and for 20–30% of those who are critically ill [3]. In a recently published meta-analysis, the pooled prevalence of AKI among all hospitalized COVID-19 patients was 28%, with 9% requiring RRT [3]. Patients of COVID-19 with AKI have a significantly worse outcome when compared to patients without AKI. Proteinuria is common in COVID-19 even without renal dysfunction and often remits spontaneously in a few weeks following clinical recovery. During the acute stage, proteinuria has been reported in 28–84% of COVID-19 patients [4]. The degree of proteinuria may vary depending on the type of glomerular involvement. Most patients have low-grade proteinuria, which can be explained due to defective reabsorption of filtered proteins seen with acute tubular injury.

Almost all cohort studies, systematic reviews, and meta-analyses have uniformly shown that CKD patients are more prone to develop severe complications of COVID-19 [5]. Apart from the chronic disease itself, the immunological state of CKD patients predisposes them to severe COVID-19. One meta-analysis with 1389 COVID-19-infected patients reported 3.03 times increased odds of developing the severe disease among CKD patients. Hypertension and diabetes mellitus per se are also associated with severe COVID-19 and being common causes of CKD in the general population; these comorbidities in tandem increase the risk of severe COVID-19 multifold [6]. Severe COVID-19 infection, in turn, has an adverse impact on the kidneys and worsens CKD progression.

9.4 COVID-19 and Kidneys: Pathophysiology and Development of Long COVID

Renal insult due to COVID-19 is multifactorial (Fig. 9.1). Severe infection and critical illness accompanying hemodynamic compromise can lead to renal dysfunction similar to that in other infections. Biopsy studies, including multiple postmortem biopsy studies, have shown acute tubular injury (ATI) as the most common histological pattern. This is followed by thrombotic microangiopathy, collapsing glomerulopathy, podocytopathy, and vasculitis-like features [7]. Though not conclusive, the SARS-CoV-2 has been demonstrated in renal biopsies, and direct viral infection is also attributed as a cause of renal injury [8]. Case reports of glomerular diseases associated with COVID-19 have been reported, but it would not be possible to attribute causation [8]. A predilection for collapsing glomerulopathy, referred to as COVAN (COVID-19-associated nephropathy) in patients with APOL1 genotype, requires further characterization. The glomerular involvement with or without podocytopathy explains the proteinuria seen in COVID-19 patients.

Post-infectious syndromes and sequelae are known with several viruses such as cytomegalovirus (CMV), Ebstein-Barr virus (EBV), chikungunya, and Coxsackie virus. Chronic fatigue syndrome, neuropsychiatric manifestations, and somatic

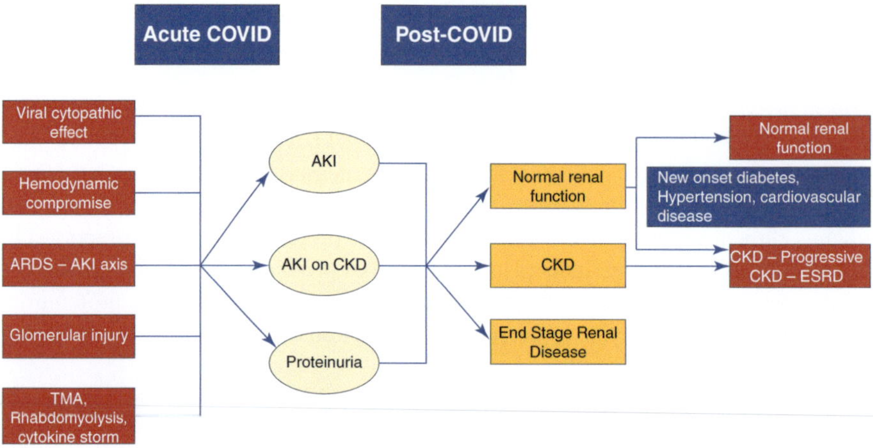

Fig. 9.1 Pathophysiology and interplay between COVID-19 and the kidney. *Footnote*: *AKI* acute kidney injury; *ARDS* acute respiratory distress syndrome; *CKD* chronic kidney disease; *ESRD* end-stage renal disease; *TMA* thrombotic microangiopathy

symptoms are common with these post-viral syndromes. This explains the biological plausibility of post-COVID-19 syndrome. A dysregulated immune system, severity of the acute infection, especially in the presence of comorbid illnesses, explains the severe manifestations and delayed/incomplete recovery seen in long COVID. Persistent renal inflammation triggers pro-fibrotic signaling and, thereby, progressive CKD is seen in a subset of long COVID patients.

9.5 Long COVID and Kidneys

Several studies have proposed the possible pathophysiologic mechanisms, direct and indirect mechanisms of nephrotoxicity, and patient outcomes in COVID-19 in these last 2 years. The primary focus of COVID-19 research after the peak COVID-19 waves has been on the long-term medical complications and sequelae of COVID-19 on multiple organ systems commonly referred to as "long COVID-19 syndrome" or "post-COVID-19 syndrome" or "post-acute sequelae of SARS-CoV-2 infection" (PASC) [9]. Long COVID is a continuum of acute illness pathogenesis (Fig. 9.2). Although up to 55 long-term effects involving almost all organ systems have been described following COVID-19 infection, renal sequelae are often more demanding with regard to the burden on healthcare resources and require special attention [10].

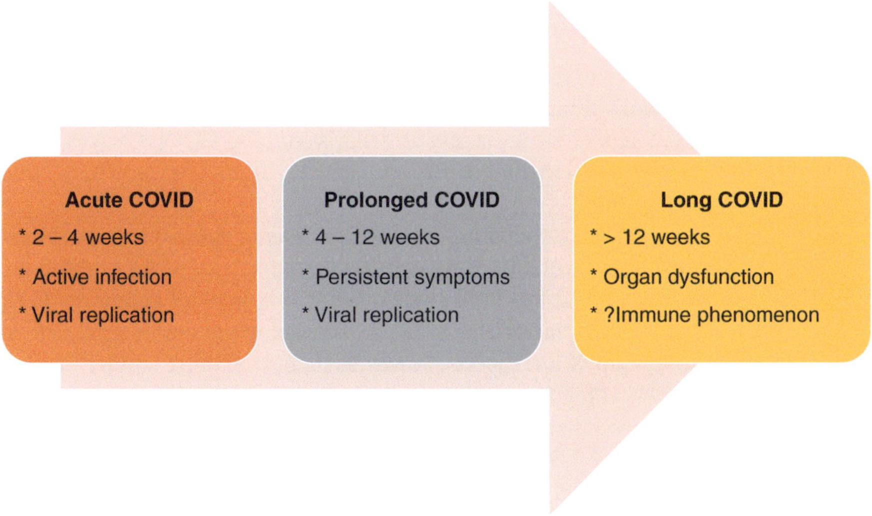

Fig. 9.2 Evolutionary phases of COVID-19 infection

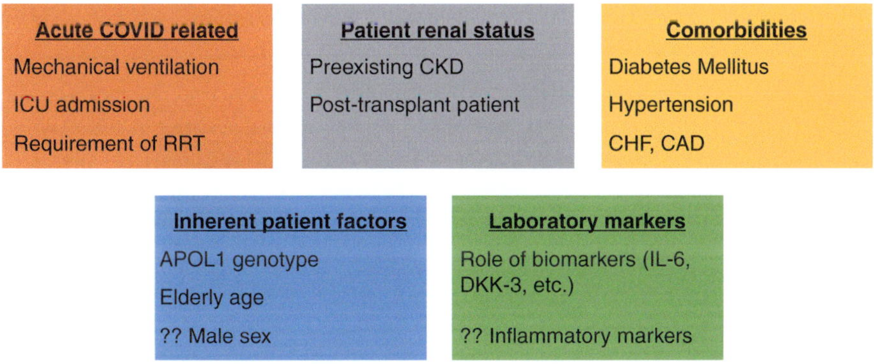

Fig. 9.3 Risk factors for kidney involvement in long COVID. *Footnote*: *APOL1* apolipoprotein L1; *CHF* congestive heart failure; *CKD* chronic kidney disease; *DKK-3* Dickkopf-3; *ICU* intensive care unit; RRT, renal replacement therapy

9.6 Risk Factors for Kidney Involvement in Long COVID

Not all patients who develop COVID-19 develop long-term complications. From the literature available, it appears that the risk of developing long COVID may depend on the severity of the acute illness and the presence of pre-existing renal disease. Though an in-depth assessment of the risk factors predisposing to long COVID involvement of the kidneys is not yet available, there are a few patient-related and disease-related risk factors that confer a higher risk for long COVID (Fig. 9.3).

9.7 Prevalence

The prevalence of long COVID is yet to be conclusively determined as several long-term studies on COVID-19 survivors are ongoing across multiple centers in the world. Moreover, the lack of clear diagnostic criteria for long COVID makes it difficult to diagnose this condition confidently and, hence, difficult to estimate its true prevalence.

Most follow-up studies showed a higher risk of persisting/new-onset renal dysfunction in COVID-19 survivors. Even patients with no evidence of AKI during the acute phase of hospitalization have reduced eGFR at 6 months of follow-up [11]. Though this can partly be explained due to the fallacies of using serum creatinine, it warrants further follow-up. Some reports, however, suggest a course similar to other influenza-like illnesses with good renal recovery in the majority of patients [12, 13]. The incidence of renal dysfunction was reported to be about 4% in the COVERSCAN cohort, a population in the UK deemed to be at low risk of COVID-19 mortality, with only 19% hospitalization rates [14]. A summary of the significant findings of renal outcomes is given in Table 9.1. There are no follow-up studies on proteinuria except one, wherein it was shown that proteinuria resolved in two-thirds of all patients by a median of 12 days, thereby suggesting a transient process [15].

Table 9.1 Renal outcomes of COVID-19 in various studies

SN	Yr.	Journal	Author	Subjects	Renal outcomes on follow-up
1	2021	*JASN*	Bowe et al. [16]	89,216 US veterans (COVID-19 survivors)	• AKI HR 1.94 (1.86–2.04) • eGFR decline ≥30% HR 1.25 (1.14–1.37) • eGFR decline ≥50% HR 1.62 (1.51–1.74) • ESKD HR 2.96 (2.49–3.51)
2	2021	*JAMA*	Nugent et al. [17]	=182 COVID-19 AKI =1430 non-COVID-19 AKI	COVID-19 AKI – decreased kidney recovery On follow-up HR 0.57 (0.35–0.92)
3	2021	*The Lancet*	Huang et al. [11]	1733	• 35% had low eGFR at 6 months of follow-up • 13% had new-onset renal dysfunction
4	2021	*JAMA*	Morin et al. [13]	478; 95 had AKI	2 patients had CKD at 4-month follow-up
5	2021	*BMJ Open*	Dennis et al. [14]	201	4% had mild renal involvement on follow-up

HR hazard ratio

9.8 Manifestations of Long COVID in Kidneys

The various long-term manifestations in the kidneys following COVID-19 are:

1. *Chronic kidney disease*—As discussed above, both new-onset and pre-existing CKD present as CKD. CKD patients and critically ill patients who received dialysis during acute COVID-19 have a higher probability of rapid progression to ESKD and need life-long renal replacement therapy. The various complications can be grouped under:
   (a) New-onset CKD
   (b) Progression of pre-existing CKD to advanced stages of CKD
   (c) End-stage kidney disease (ESKD)
2. *Glomerular disease*—Proteinuria is commonly reported in COVID-19-affected patients during the acute phase. In most cases, proteinuria is transient due to acute illness and cannot be solely attributed to SARS-CoV-2. Significant and persistent proteinuria is seen when the glomerular filtration barrier is affected and can be due to podocytopathy, COVAN (especially in African Americans with APOL1 genotype), and also thrombotic microangiopathy [4].
3. Case reports of ANCA vasculitis, IgA vasculitis, lupus, and anti-GBM disease in patients with COVID-19—These are less likely to remit unless treated with directed immunosuppressive therapies and may progress to CKD [8].

9.9 COVID-19 and Renal Transplantation

Renal transplant recipients constitute a distinctive group of kidney patients who need long-term immunosuppression for stable kidney function. This makes them predisposed to COVID-19 (and severe COVID-19). The lack of a specific antiviral therapy necessitated multiple therapies like hydroxychloroquine, ivermectin, remdesivir, tocilizumab, and protease inhibitors-based anti-retroviral therapies (lopinavir/ritonavir) in the management of COVID-19 [18]. Remdesivir has been used successfully in transplant recipients without significant adverse effects [19]. Apart from the uncertain efficacy, the use of protease inhibitors which inhibit CYP3A metabolism results in significant calcineurin inhibitor (tacrolimus and cyclosporine) toxicity and precludes their use in transplant recipients [18]. Considering their immunosuppressed state with multiple comorbidities, they are expected to have delayed recovery after COVID-19. In one study involving transplant recipients, only 11.53% of COVID-19 survivors were free of clinical symptoms or laboratory abnormality during routine follow-up evaluation [20]. Also, these abnormalities depend on a history of hospitalization, presence of diabetes mellitus, and degree of renal function (eGFR) in the post-COVID-19 period in these patients. The coagulation abnormalities, in particular, were more frequent in these patients.

In addition to the above mentioned clinical outcomes, immunological outcomes are of particular concern in this patient population. COVID-19 infection necessitates modification of maintenance immunosuppressive regimen in most transplant recipients. This increases the risk of organ rejection. Furthermore, change in immunoreactivity against alloantigens due to SARS-CoV-2 and persistent immunoreactivity to the virus during follow-up is reported. The B-cell and T-cell response to antigens and immunosuppressive drugs after COVID-19 is unclear. The clinical implications of these findings about the risk of graft rejection and/or future risk of malignancy as seen with other immunomodulatory viruses like CMV, EBV, or BKV needs to be evaluated on follow-up.

9.10 Screening

All patients who have recovered from COVID-19 need to be evaluated post-discharge for features of long COVID. An ideal post-COVID-19 care clinic needs multidisciplinary collaboration between pulmonologists, general physicians, physiotherapists, specialist nurses, psychological counselors, researchers, and support groups to ensure complete recovery. One such initiative which has shown positive results is the RECOVERY program, a comprehensive post-COVID-19 center at Yale [21]. In resource-limited settings, teleconsultation can be done for recovered patients to identify those at risk for long COVID, and those patients can be subsequently evaluated in detail in the clinic. General screening of all recovered patients should include a blood pressure measurement and blood sugar estimation. New-onset hypertension and diabetes have also been reported in COVID-19 survivors, and these, in turn, increase the risk for progressive CKD [22, 23].

For patients with suspected kidney involvement, the following investigations are suggested:

1. Urine routine and microscopy
2. Blood urea and serum creatinine
3. Urine protein/creatinine ratio
4. Hemogram
5. Ultrasonography of kidneys

All patients with new-onset renal dysfunction and progressive CKD need to be evaluated to rule out other common causes of worsening renal function. If clinically indicated, an autoimmune workup, serum protein electrophoresis, urine sediment evaluation, and advanced imaging studies must be performed.

Standard renal function tests are considered late markers and are deranged only after the injury is established. The search for renal troponin has been ongoing for decades. Tubular injury is most common in COVID-19, and tubular biomarkers have been evaluated for this purpose. One such marker, Dickkopf-3 (DKK-3), when expressed, increases the risk of tubulointerstitial fibrosis. Following tubular injury, urinary DKK-3 and interleukin-6 (IL-6) increase in the acute phase due to tubular injury and inflammation. Studies have shown that if they remain elevated at 6 months, or demonstrate a biphasic increase after the initial fall in levels, this indicates fibroblast activation, abnormal cytokine signaling, and propensity to progressive fibrosis [24]. Larger prospective studies of biomarkers are needed to understand their role in monitoring the AKI–CKD transition in COVID-19 survivors.

9.11 Management

The natural history of long COVID is still largely unknown. Also, with no known preventive drugs and/or strategies for long COVID, optimal medical management remains the only option. Because of limited evidence, definitive management recommendations have not been published. Most of the management protocols rely on local clinical experience and prior data from influenza-like illnesses and consensus guidelines. Renal function tests of COVID-19 survivors have to be monitored periodically after recovery. Any patient with a rapid progression, defined as a yearly eGFR decrease >5 mL/min/1.73m^2, will need re-evaluation for other confounding factors. If there are no other apparent causes, general management of CKD is to be done. A comprehensive renal care plan consisting of regular monitoring of renal function in consultation with the nephrologist is essential.

Medical management is the cornerstone of therapy in CKD patients. Apart from COVID-19-related inflammation, multiple factors may affect kidney disease progression [25]. Blood pressure and glycemic control have to be ensured to slow down the progression of kidney failure. Though there were initial speculations about the harmful effects of angiotensin-converting enzyme inhibitors (ACEi) in COVID-19 patients, subsequent well-conducted randomized studies have failed to show any risk of adverse effects with the use of these drugs. ACEi and angiotensin receptor blockers (ARBs) remain the drug of choice for the management of hypertension with appropriate monitoring for hyperkalemia. The utility of steroids, anticoagulants, and/or other drugs in long COVID is being evaluated in multiple prospective and randomized trials worldwide.

Complications of kidney disease are often evident after stage 3 CKD and necessitate specific therapy. Management of anemia with iron supplementation and erythropoietin-stimulating agents (if hemoglobin <10 g/dL), bicarbonate supplementation for acidosis, and vitamin D therapy for mineral bone disease need to be optimized. Dialysis access planning in advanced CKD (stage 4/5) should be done. Patients with CKD are more susceptible to cardiovascular diseases. COVID-19 survivors also have an increased risk of cardiovascular disease. Therefore the risk factors are additive and a comprehensive cardiovascular assessment has to be performed.

9.12 Conclusion

Renal involvement in COVID-19 has been recognized from the beginning of the pandemic and our understanding has evolved significantly. Nevertheless, further research is required to identify potential modifying factors, genetic predisposition as in APOL1 genotype, biomarkers to detect and monitor the renal injury, and disease-modifying therapy for COVID-19. Collaborative studies like the National COVID Cohort Collaborative (N3C) will help us to evaluate the long-term clinical consequences comprehensively and generate COVID-19 analytics for better informed patient care and follow-up [26]. Comprehensive post-COVID-19 programs and clinics will play an important role not only for patient care but also to carry out research that will help us better manage COVID-19 survivors. As our understanding of COVID-19 evolves, our management plan for post-COVID-19 survivors is bound to change with time.

9.13 Take-Home Points

- Kidney patients are more susceptible to acquiring COVID-19 infection and developing severe illness.
- Case definition of long COVID-19 syndrome requires standardization to allow valid diagnosis and establish management strategies.
- Long-COVID in kidneys can manifest as CKD, ESRD, or glomerular disease.
- Patients with severe COVID-19, AKI, and/or proteinuria during acute COVID-19 and patients with CKD who had COVID-19 need regular monitoring of renal function after discharge.
- Any new, persistent, or progressive renal dysfunction/proteinuria needs assessment by a nephrologist.
- General management of hypertension, diabetes, and CKD with closer follow-up for those with ongoing renal issues is paramount.

References

1. Heung M, Chawla LS. Acute kidney injury: gateway to chronic kidney disease. Nephron Clin Pract. 2014 Sep 24;127(1–4):30–4.
2. Chapter 1: Definition and classification of CKD. Kidney Int Suppl. 2013 Jan;3(1):19–62.
3. Silver SA, Beaubien-Souligny W, Shah PS, et al. The prevalence of acute kidney injury in patients hospitalized with COVID-19 infection: a systematic review and meta-analysis. Kidney Med. 2021 Feb;3(1):83–98.e1.
4. Mohamed MMB, Velez JCQ. Proteinuria in COVID-19. Clin Kidney J. 2021 Mar 1;14(Supplement_1):i40–7.
5. Long JD, Strohbehn I, Sawtell R, et al. COVID-19 survival and its impact on chronic kidney disease. Transl Res J Lab Clin Med. 2021 Nov 10;S1931-5244(21):00266–8.
6. Callender LA, Curran M, Bates SM, et al. The impact of pre-existing co-morbidities and therapeutic interventions on COVID-19. Front Immunol. 2020;11:1991.

7. Sharma P, Ng JH, Bijol V, et al. Pathology of COVID-19-associated acute kidney injury. Clin Kidney J. 2021 Mar 1;14(Supplement_1):i30–9.
8. Shimmel A, Shaikhouni S, Mariani L. Current understanding of clinical manifestations of COVID-19 in glomerular disease. Glomerular Dis. 2021;1(4):250–64.
9. Nalbandian A, Sehgal K, Gupta A, et al. Post-acute COVID-19 syndrome. Nat Med. 2021 Apr;27(4):601–15.
10. Lopez-Leon S, Wegman-Ostrosky T, Perelman C, et al. More than 50 long-term effects of COVID-19: a systematic review and meta-analysis. Sci Rep. 2021 Aug 9;11(1):16144.
11. Huang C, Huang L, Wang Y, et al. 6-month consequences of COVID-19 in patients discharged from hospital: a cohort study. Lancet. 2021 Jan 16;397(10270):220–32.
12. Bouquegneau A, Huart J, Lutteri L, et al. POS-196 patients with covid-19 mostly recover from tubular proteinuria and acute kidney injury after hospital discharge. Kidney Int Rep. 2021 Apr 1;6(4):S82.
13. Writing Committee for the COMEBAC Study Group, Morin L, Savale L, Pham T, et al. Four-month clinical status of a cohort of patients after hospitalization for COVID-19. JAMA. 2021 Apr 20;325(15):1525–34.
14. Dennis A, Wamil M, Alberts J, et al. Multiorgan impairment in low-risk individuals with post-COVID-19 syndrome: a prospective, community-based study. BMJ Open. 2021 Mar 30;11(3):e048391.
15. Pei G, Zhang Z, Peng J, et al. Renal involvement and early prognosis in patients with COVID-19 pneumonia. J Am Soc Nephrol JASN. 2020 Jun;31(6):1157–65.
16. Bowe B, Xie Y, Xu E, Al-Aly Z. Kidney outcomes in Long COVID. J Am Soc Nephrol JASN. 2021 Nov;32(11):2851–62.
17. Nugent J, Aklilu A, Yamamoto Y, et al. Assessment of acute kidney injury and longitudinal kidney function after hospital discharge among patients with and without COVID-19. JAMA Netw Open. 2021 Mar 1;4(3):e211095.
18. Kataria A, Yakubu I, Winstead R, et al. COVID-19 in kidney transplantation: epidemiology, management considerations, and the impact on kidney transplant practice. Transplant Direct. 2020 Aug;6(8):e582.
19. Meshram HS, Kute VB, Patel H, et al. Feasibility and safety of remdesivir in SARS-CoV2 infected renal transplant recipients: a retrospective cohort from a developing nation. Transpl Infect Dis. 2021 Aug;23(4):e13629.
20. Basic-Jukic N, Juric I, Furic-Cunko V, et al. Follow-up of renal transplant recipients after acute COVID-19—a prospective cohort single-center study. Immun Inflamm Dis. 2021;9(4):1563–72.
21. Lutchmansingh DD, Knauert MP, Antin-Ozerkis DE, et al. A clinic blueprint for post-coronavirus disease 2019 recovery: learning from the past. Looking to the Future Chest. 2021 Mar;159(3):949–58.
22. Ayoubkhani D, Khunti K, Nafilyan V, et al. Post-covid syndrome in individuals admitted to hospital with covid-19: retrospective cohort study. BMJ. 2021 Mar;31(372):n693.
23. Chen G, Li X, Gong Z, et al. Hypertension as a sequela in patients of SARS-CoV-2 infection. PLoS One. 2021 Apr 28;16(4):e0250815.
24. Husain Syed F, Villa G, Wilhelm J, et al. Renal markers for monitoring acute kidney injury transition to chronic kidney disease after COVID-19. Nephrol Dial Transplant. 2021 Nov 1;36(11):2143–7.
25. Yende S, Parikh CR. Long COVID and kidney disease. Nat Rev Nephrol. 2021 Dec;17(12):792–3.
26. Haendel MA, Chute CG, Bennett TD, et al. The national COVID cohort collaborative (N3C): rationale, design, infrastructure, and deployment. J Am Med Inform Assoc. 2021 Mar 1;28(3):427–43.

10 COVID-19 Sequelae Affecting Ear, Nose and Throat

Alok Thakar, Smriti Panda, and Kapil Sikka

10.1 Introduction

Otorhinolaryngologic (ENT) manifestations have been recognized as salient features of SARS-CoV-2 infection since the beginning of the COVID-19 pandemic [1]. These symptoms from the upper aerodigestive tract were predominant in the subset of COVID-19 patients presenting with mild to moderate symptomatology [2]. In a large study performed on 225 patients affected with mild COVID-19 from a tertiary care center in India, at least 1 ENT symptom was identified in 62.2% of the study population [2]. The most commonly reported symptom was odynophagia (63.5%) followed by smell and taste disturbances (20% overall and 46.8% of ENT manifestations). These results were comparable with the outcomes reported in a recently concluded systematic review and meta-analysis [3].

As the pandemic evolved, it was observed that certain ENT manifestations persisted even after a patient was deemed to have been cured of COVID-19 [4, 5]. These manifestations, therefore, fall under the spectrum of post-COVID-19 sequelae, if duration of symptoms persists beyond 12 weeks from the diagnosis of COVID-19 [6]. Certain upper aerodigestive tract symptoms also emerged in patients following COVID-19 recovery that could be attributed to therapeutic interventions directed toward COVID-19 or immunological origin secondary to COVID-19 rather than a true manifestation of post-COVID-19 sequelae [7–9]. Figure 10.1 depicts the wide array of ENT manifestations reported in literature persisting beyond the diagnosis of COVID-19. This chapter will discuss the ENT manifestations in light of post-COVID-19 sequelae emphasizing pathophysiology and evidence-based management.

A. Thakar · S. Panda (✉) · K. Sikka
Department of Otorhinolaryngology, AIIMS, New Delhi, India

A. Mohan, S. Mittal (eds.), *Post COVID-19 Complications and Management*,
https://doi.org/10.1007/978-981-19-4407-9_10

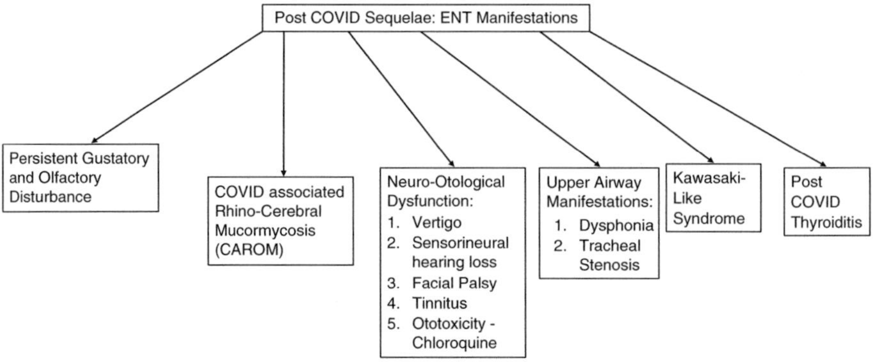

Fig. 10.1 Spectrum of ENT manifestations described in association with post-COVID-19 sequelae

10.2 Smell and Taste Disturbances

10.2.1 Epidemiology

Gustatory and olfactory disturbances have long been recognized as sequelae of viral illness. The viruses implicated include rhinovirus, parainfluenza virus, and Epstein-Barr virus [10, 11]. Anosmia (complete loss of smell) has a reported incidence of 1% globally [12]. Of these, post-infectious olfactory dysfunction (PIOD) accounts for 11% of the cases and 20–30% in high-volume referral centers [12–14]. COVID-19 as a contributor to PIOD revealed some interesting characteristics. Various degrees of smell and taste disturbances have been reported during the course of the illness. In a large multicentric European study involving patients with mild to moderate symptomatology, smell and taste disturbances were reported in 85.6% and 88%, respectively [15]. A systematic review and meta-analysis investigating possible ethnic differences in the smell and taste disturbances revealed a pooled incidence rate of 47.4% for combined olfactory and taste disturbance [16]. This study identified lower incidence rates in studies reported from Asia (17.7%) compared to Europe (54.8%). Apart from contributing to chemosensory loss in a large proportion of individuals, olfactory and gustatory disturbances were noted to be the sentinel symptom in 25% of patients in the study performed by Kaye et al. using the "Anosmia Reporting Tool" [17]. Studies using patient-reported outcomes and questionnaires reported lower incidence rates than studies utilizing objective smell identification tools as the former was prone to recall bias [16]. Given the disease burden of COVID-19 infectivity and the preponderance of chemosensory dysfunction in infected individuals, an estimated incidence of 20 million individuals has been drawn to have perceived some degree of chemosensory dysfunction [18].

10.2.2 Natural History of COVID-19 Chemosensory Dysfunction

In the multicentric European study, the overall early recovery rate was to the tune of 44% [15]. Of all affected persons, 72.6% recovered their smell and taste disturbance within 8 days. In the study conducted on mild COVID-19 patients from India, 96% of patients had recovered completely at 4 weeks [2]. These studies reflect the overall reversibility and excellent prognosis of COVID-19 chemosensory dysfunction. There is a lack of evidence about the true incidence of long-standing PIOD following COVID-19. Vaira and colleagues prospectively evaluated 138 patients diagnosed with COVID-19 to elucidate long-term recovery rates of chemosensory dysfunction [19]. They found that 7.2% of patients had persistent severe PIOD 60 days from the day of diagnosis of COVID-19. Continued dysfunction for smell at 20 days and continued taste dysfunction at 10 days were risk factors for persistent PIOD. This provided an insight into the possibility of initiating therapeutic strategies during this critical window period.

10.2.3 Reinfection Anosmia

Lechien et al. have reported two cases of chemosensory dysfunction occurring in the reinfection to COVID-19 setting in individuals who had previously experienced similar dysfunction and had fully recovered from it [20].

Favorable indicators toward the recovery of long-standing chemosensory dysfunction include the following:

(a) The appearance of parosmia [21].
(b) Olfactory bulb (OB) volume determined on coronal T2-weighted MRI revealing a volume of 40 cc for one olfactory bulb is generally indicative of recovery [22].

10.2.4 Pathophysiology

1. *Obstruction of nasal airflow*: This theory is the most frequent explanation for non-COVID-19 PIOD, especially during the acute phase of viral infection [10]. Viruses causing upper respiratory tract infection typically induce inflammation and edema of the nasal mucosa resulting in obstruction to transport of odorants to the olfactory epithelium. This variety of PIOD reverses as and when inflammation subsides. This mechanism is unlikely to be the basis for the widely reported COVID-19-induced PIOD because symptoms of nasal mucosal inflammation are infrequent in COVID-19 [23].
2. *Virus-induced destruction of olfactory neuron and epithelium*: This theory again explains PIOD in the non-COVID-19 settings, especially those cases where

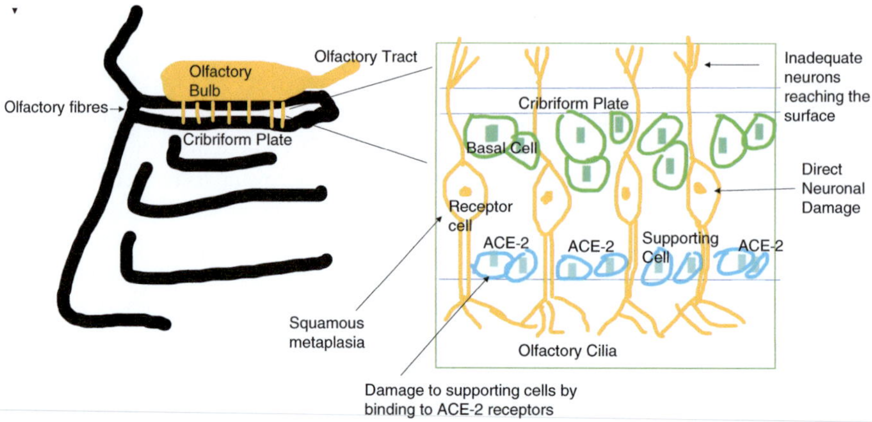

Fig. 10.2 Schematic representation of mechanism behind virus-induced chemosensory disturbance

there is permanent chemosensory dysfunction (Fig. 10.2). Histopathological studies and animal models have provided great insight into the pathophysiology of virus-induced PIOD:

(a) There is ultrastructural evidence of direct neuronal injury induced by a viral infection, in the form of partial loss of neurons, disorganized epithelium with reduced olfactory receptor cells, nerve bundles, and squamous metaplasia [24].
(b) There is inadequate number of neurons that reach the epithelial surface, thereby not coming in contact with the odor stimulant [25].
(c) In a mouse model of COVID-19, extensive damage of olfactory epithelium was identified by Bryche et al. This resulted in the exposure of olfactory neurons. The virus could be isolated from the epithelium at day 2 and the viral load gradually reduced till day 4. However, the virus could not be demonstrated in the olfactory bulb or cortex [26].

Though this theory holds for non-COVID-19 PIOD, its relevance in COVID-19-induced PIOD is questionable. This is due to the absence of ACE-2 and TMPRSS2 receptors in olfactory neurons. The presence of these receptors serves as portals for the entry of SARS-CoV-2 [27].

3. *Virus-induced damage of sustentacular cells in the olfactory epithelium*:
Unlike olfactory neurons, the sustentacular cells in the olfactory epithelium harbor ACE-2 and TMPRSS2 receptors. Bilinska et al. have proposed the mechanism for COVID-19-induced PIOD resulting from virus-induced destruction of sustentacular cells [27].

10.2.5 Diagnostic Work-Up

Detailed evaluation protocol is available in Table 10.1.

Table 10.1 Suggested work-up for post-infectious olfactory disturbance

Work-up strategy	Description
History	• Detailed history: onset, duration; specifics of impairment, qualitative or quantitative, accompanying gustatory impairment, effect on quality of life • Identify red flags: neurological symptoms, unilateral nasal obstruction, persistent headache, weight loss
ENT examination	• Endoscopic evaluation: rigid or flexible endoscope • Visualize olfactory cleft • Identify inflammatory conditions • Identify space-occupying lesions obstructing airflow toward olfactory cleft
Imaging	• NCCT PNS: opacification of olfactory cleft. Rule out inflammatory and neoplastic conditions • MRI brain and PNS: T2-weighted sequence to evaluate olfactory bulb area (volume, sulcus depth). Volumetric assessment of olfactory eloquent areas
Olfactory testing	
Subjective patient-reported outcomes	• Examples: visual analogue scale, questionnaire for olfactory dysfunction • To be used in conjunction with objective testing • Ideal for monitoring response to intervention
Psychophysical testing	Components of olfactory testing: • Odor threshold: lowest concentration of the odorant perceived by the patient. Does not require odor identification • Odor discrimination: ability to differentiate between the odors • Odor identification: ability to correctly name the odorant being presented Commercially available kits: • Sniffin' Sticks test • Smell diskettes • UPSIT (University of Pennsylvania Smell Identification Test) • Connecticut Chemosensory Clinical Research Centre Test • Toyota and Takagi olfactometer • U-Sniff • European retronasal test
Objective functional testing	• Olfactory event-related potentials • Functional MRI

Essential components of diagnostic work-up include [18]:

- *Nasal endoscopy*: Conductive pathologies impairing nasal airflow in the region of the olfactory cleft need to be ruled out before diagnosing PIOD.
- *Subjective patient-reported questionnaires*: Table 10.1 enumerates the various validated structured patient-reported questionnaires available for olfactory and gustatory function evaluation.
- *Psychophysical testing*: This involves presenting an olfactory stimulant and recording the patient's outcome. A detailed description of psychophysical testing is provided in Table 10.1. The integral components include:

  - Odor threshold
  - Odor discrimination
  - Odor identification
- *Electrophysiology*: This involves presenting odor stimuli and recording event potentials from recording electrodes placed in the olfactory epithelium (electro-olfactogram).
- *Imaging*: T2-weighted coronal MRI of the paranasal sinus and brain should be performed to evaluate the following parameters:
  - Olfactory bulb volume
  - Olfactory sulcus depth
  - Volumetric assessment of olfactory eloquent regions of the brain
  - To identify pathologies interfering with airflow to the olfactory cleft: polyp, septal deviation, space-occupying lesions, chronic rhinosinusitis, and turbinate hypertrophy

In non-contrast CT of paranasal sinuses, opacification of olfactory cleft also correlates well with olfactory disturbance post-COVID-19 [28].

Functional MRI: This modality provides a dynamic assessment of olfaction-associated cortical activity. fMRI facility is not easily available, and hence, the use of this modality should be restricted to clinical trials and research purposes.

10.2.6 Management

Table 10.2 summarizes the various therapeutic interventions reported in the literature for COVID-19-induced chemosensory dysfunction.

The Cochrane Library has initiated a live systematic review and meta-analysis to identify randomized trials for the prevention of COVID-19-induced prolonged PIOD [29] and has identified only one randomized controlled trial. Abdelalim et al. randomized patients with less than 4 weeks of olfactory disturbance to receive either topical nasal corticosteroids (mometasone furoate) or no treatment (both groups received additional olfactory training) [30]. No statistically significant difference was noted between the two groups on serial follow-up. The authors concluded the lack of superiority of topical steroid therapy over and above olfactory training.

10.2.7 Olfactory Training

Olfactory training involves regular presentation of standardized formulation of olfactory stimulants to the participants, who in turn are encouraged to focus on the memory of the odor being presented. Presumed mechanisms of action include reorganization of the olfactory epithelium, olfactory bulb, and neural olfactory pathway [29].

Table 10.2 Summary of potential therapeutic options for COVID-19-induced PIOD

Treatment strategy	Salient features
Conservative management	• One-third of patients with PIOD recover spontaneously Rate of recovery: degree of initial loss, patient age, and duration of loss
Smoking cessation	Degree of olfactory dysfunction is greater with ongoing smoking. Therefore, smoking cessation should be encouraged
Olfactory training	Robust evidence available favoring olfactory training strategies in recovery of PIOD
Corticosteroids	• Poor quality of evidence in non-COVID-19 PIOD • No consensus on oral versus intranasal steroid, dose, and frequency of administration Paucity of evidence in COVID-19-associated PIOD. Individualized risk-benefit assessment should be taken into consideration prior to initiating oral steroids • Intranasal steroid administered by Kaiteki technique improves bioavailability at the level of olfactory cleft
Theophylline	• Inhibit phosphodiesterase and increase cyclic AMP • Assists in neuroepithelium regeneration • Existing evidence insufficient to guide its use in PIOD
Sodium citrate	• Intranasal route • Ability to sequester calcium ions, reducing free mucosal calcium, inhibiting negative feedback loop, and increasing sensitivity to odorant • Mixed results in its efficacy in non-COVID-19 PIOD
N-methyl-D-aspartate antagonist	• Caroverine • Inhibiting olfactory bulb feedback mechanism • Requires well-designed RCT to determine efficacy in COVID-19 PIOD
Alpha lipoic acid	• Stimulates expression of nerve growth factors: substance P, neuropeptide Y • Neuroprotective effect • Moderate improvement in olfaction in non-COVID-19 PIOD
Vitamin A	• Regeneration of neuroepithelium • Studies have explored systemic as well as intranasal vitamin A
Minocycline	• Anti-apoptotic agent • No proven benefit in PIOD
Zinc sulfate	No available evidence favoring the use of zinc sulfate in improving olfactory function in PIOD

1. Classic Olfactory Training: This therapy involves 5 min exposure of four odorants twice a day: phenyl ethyl alcohol, eucalyptol, citronella, and eugenol. The duration of therapy is for 12 weeks.
2. Modified Olfactory Training: This variant of olfactory training is divided into three parts, each consisting of 12 weeks of therapy as described above:

   12 weeks: Twice a day 5-min exposure of phenyl ethyl alcohol, eucalyptol, citronella, and eugenol

   12 weeks: The above regime is followed by another 2 weeks of therapy with 5 min twice a day exposure of menthol, thyme, tangerine, and jasmine.

12 weeks: The last 12 weeks comprise exposure to green tea, bergamot, rosemary, and gardenia

Pekala et al. and Sorokowska et al. have independently demonstrated the benefit of the above intervention in the pre-COVID-19 era by their systematic review and meta-analysis [31, 32].

10.2.8 Role of Steroids

In a recently concluded review, significant heterogeneity was noted in studies evaluating the role of steroids in PIOD in terms of formulation, route of administration, and dosage [18]. The action of steroids in PIOD is mainly in reducing the inflammatory component of olfactory dysfunction rather than any beneficial effect on the olfactory neuroepithelium [18]. At present, there is no clarity whether oral or topical formulation should be preferred in the case of post-COVID-19 PIOD. The other issue plaguing the studies conducted on the role of steroids in COVID-19 PIOD is the confounding factor of rampant steroid administration in cases of moderate to severe COVID-19 as well as in post-COVID-19 sequelae. Currently, there is no robust indicator to administer oral corticosteroids for chemosensory dysfunction following COVID-19. Many studies have revealed the promising role of topical steroids, provided they are administered accurately to deliver the drug to the olfactory cleft [33, 34]. Kaiteki position has been advocated for improving the bioavailability of topical steroids at the level of the olfactory cleft [35]. This involves lying down on one side with the extension of the chin and neck in an upward direction. Kaiteki position increases steroid availability to olfactory cleft by 96% in the decongested nose and 75% in the non-decongested nose [35].

10.3 Phantosmia

Phantosmia or olfactory hallucination has been described in the background of COVID-19. Compared to the chemosensory dysfunction described above, reports of phantosmia are restricted to anecdotal reports [36].

10.4 COVID-19-Associated Rhino-Orbito-Cerebral Mucormycosis (CAROM)

10.4.1 Etiopathogenesis

The causative agent behind the pathogenesis of acute invasive fungal sinusitis belongs to the order Mucorales, followed by *Aspergillus* species. The species most commonly isolated is *Rhizopus oryzae*. The other less commonly reported species include *Mucor*, *Absidia*, and *Cunninghamella* [37]. These fungal pathogens are ubiquitous in the environment and result in fulminant sinusitis in a susceptible host in the presence of suitable environmental conditions favoring its growth (tropical climate and high humidity) [38]. The host factors responsible for the development of acute invasive mucormycosis are as follows [39]:

- Uncontrolled diabetes mellitus
- Steroid use
- Post-organ transplant immunosuppression
- Retroviral disease
- Hematological malignancy
- Malnutrition
- Severe burns
- Long-term chemotherapy

The hallmark clinical features of acute invasive rhino-orbito-cerebral mucormycosis (ROCM) have been described by Smith and Kirchner et al. in 1950 [40] (Fig. 10.3):

- Black, necrotic turbinate associated with nasal crusting and blood-tinged nasal discharge
- Characteristic facial pain with or without paresthesia along the second division of trigeminal nerve (early sign)
- Periorbital or peri-nasal swelling with or without discoloration or blackening
- Orbital symptoms: ptosis, proptosis, vision loss, and complete ophthalmoplegia
- Multiple cranial neuropathies—rapid onset. Cranial neuropathy may be unrelated to the clinically apparent disease extension

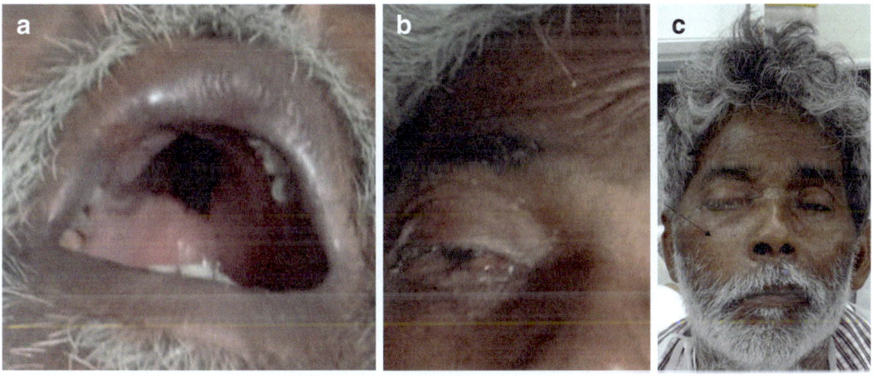

Fig. 10.3 Clinical features of CAROM. (**a**) Black eschar formation over the palate. (**b**) Complete ophthalmoplegia, vision loss, and chemosis signifying cavernous sinus involvement. (**c**) Disease extension to premaxillary soft tissue presenting as cheek fullness (arrow)

The constellation of symptoms described above in the background of a susceptible host should prompt the clinician to consider the possibility of ROCM.

ROCM most commonly presents with sinonasal involvement (88.9%) followed by orbital and cavernous sinus extension (56.7%) and intracranial involvement (22.2%) [41]. Talmi et al. have proposed a staging system for ROCM with discriminative power in terms of survival outcome [42]:

- Stage I—disease localized to the nose only with minimal soft tissue invasion (100% survival)
- Stage II—disease limited to the nose, ipsilateral sinus, and orbit (80% survival)
- Stage III—disease extending to intracranial structures with unimpaired or minimal impairment of cognition (67% survival)
- Stage IV—disease involving intracranial structures with impaired consciousness or hemiplegia, bilateral disease, skin necrosis, and palatal involvement (0% survival)

10.4.2 ROCM in the Background of COVID-19: CAROM

The second wave of the COVID-19 pandemic in India witnessed a dramatic surge in the incidence of ROCM. The pre-pandemic incidence of ROCM has been 0.14/1000 population which is 80 times higher than the incidence quoted from western literature [43]. However, the second wave-associated ROCM resulted in 14,872 cases being reported as of May 28, 2021 [44]. The salient features of CAROM are summarized as follows:

- CAROM has been described as both synchronous with the detection of COVID-19 and after recovery from the viral illness. On an average, CAROM developed 17.6 days following the onset of COVID-19. This time period was longer, with cases being reported 4–5 weeks from the onset of COVID-19 toward the beginning of the CAROM wave [45].
- The predominant comorbid condition associated with CAROM was uncontrolled diabetes mellitus, with few studies quoting 100% association. About 70% of the patients had a documented blood glucose level greater than 300 mg/dl at presentation [46]. A systematic review reported a pooled incidence of concomitant ketoacidosis to be 14.9% [41].
- The same systematic review identified steroid usage in 76.3% CAROM cases [41]. Nevertheless, CAROM was predominantly reported in patients with mild to moderate disease rather than severe COVID-19 illness [47]. According to the report from AIIMS, New Delhi, CAROM was associated with mild COVID-19 in 54%, moderate disease in 33%, and severe disease in 13%, respectively [48].
- CAROM is a fulminant disease with time to initiation of treatment having a direct bearing on survival outcomes. Time-sensitive initiation of surgical debridement and antifungal therapy can have a tremendous impact on prognosis. The

mortality rate of CAROM ranges from 33 to 80%. A delay of 6 days in the initiation of treatment can double the incidence of 30-day mortality [49].
- Survival is found to be higher in patients who undergo complete surgical debridement along with timely initiation of antifungal treatment (64.9%) versus patients who only receive antifungal treatment (21.73%) [7].

10.4.3 Pathogenesis of CAROM

Figure 10.4 depicts the complex interplay of various factors unique to COVID-19 that predisposes an individual to CAROM:

- *Role of ACE-2 receptors*: Since there is generalized upregulation of ACE-2 receptors in COVID-19, the upregulation in pancreatic islet cells causes insulin resistance [50].
- *Concomitant uncontrolled diabetes mellitus*: Hyperglycemia and the acidic pH associated with the development of ketoacidosis in the background of COVID-19-induced hypoxia provide an ideal substrate for the growth of mucormycosis. Hyperglycemia upregulates the expression of glucose-regulator protein 78 (GRP-78) of endothelium cells and fungal ligand spore coating homolog (CotH) protein. This facilitates angioinvasion, hematogenous dissemination, and tissue necrosis [41, 51].
- *Neutrophil and T cell dysfunction*: COVID-19 infection dysregulates the balance between CD-4 and CD-8 T cells and reduces CD-4 lymphocyte-induced gamma

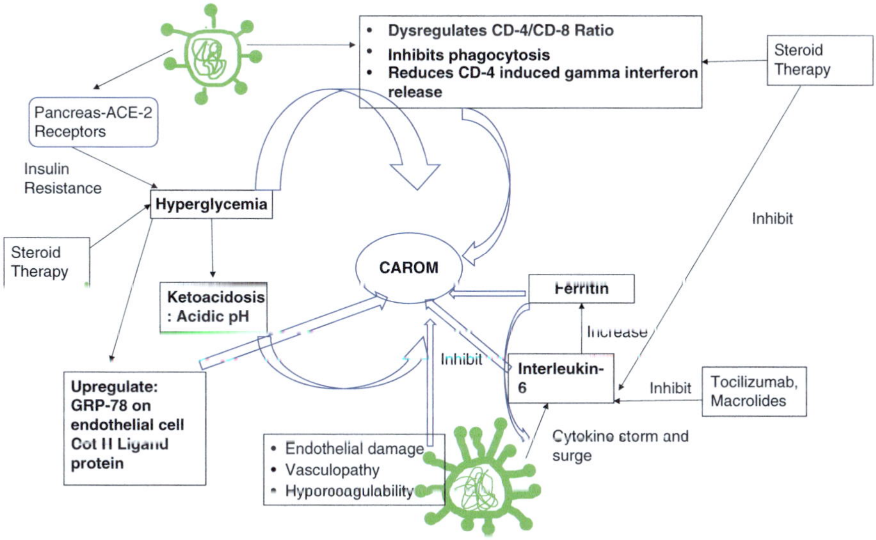

Fig. 10.4 Pathogenesis of CAROM

interferon release, thereby blunting phagocytic response against opportunistic bacterial and fungal infection [52].

- *Role of steroid therapy*: The role of steroid therapy has been widely investigated. Glucocorticoids are known to give rise to a hyperglycemic state. Glucocorticoids also interfere with phagocytic function by inhibiting pro-inflammatory cytokines like IL-6 and inhibiting phagocytosis [47].
- *Role of IL-6*: Interleukin-6 plays the role of a double-edged sword. COVID-19, a pro-inflammatory state, is associated with a surge of IL-6 levels (cytokine storm). IL-6, in turn, interferes with iron metabolism by increasing ferritin levels. Very high ferritin levels perpetuate the pro-inflammatory cascade and provide excellent conditions for mucormycosis to thrive and perpetuate the disease process. High ferritin levels also induce iron-free radical-induced oxidative damage [53]. However, IL-6 is known to mount an immune response against opportunistic infection. Use of steroid and IL-6 inhibitor tocilizumab interferes with IL-6-induced phagocytic property, thereby predisposing to opportunistic fungal infection [54]. Macrolide antibiotics like azithromycin, which were frequently administered to COVID-19 patients, are also known to inhibit IL-6 production [55].
- *Role of serum ferritin*: Increased ferritin levels seen in COVID-19 infection owing to a pro-inflammatory state predispose to the development of ROCM as Mucorales thrive in an environment rich in iron [41].
- *Hypercoagulopathy and vasculitis*: COVID-19 is known to be associated with immune-mediated vasculopathy and cause direct endothelial damage. This can compound the angioinvasive manifestation of mucormycosis, for example, the development of CRAO (central retinal artery occlusion) [45].
- *Role of zinc*: The role of zinc was investigated in vitro by comparing the growth of *Mucor* in zinc-enriched and zinc-depleted media, with the former showing growth favoring *Mucor* [56]. However, serum levels of zinc were not found to be different among patients with CAROM and COVID-19 patients without ROCM.

10.4.4 Diagnosis

The following laboratory investigations can render the confirmatory diagnosis of CAROM:

- KOH mount: This is a bedside investigation where nasal crust or tissue from necrotic areas is subjected to microscopy under 10% KOH mount [57]. The presence of septate hyphae indicates the possibility of *Aspergillus* species, whereas aseptate hyphae are pathognomic of *Mucorales* species.
- Imaging: The reasons for obtaining cross-sectional radiology are the following (Fig. 10.5):
  - To confirm the diagnosis of CAROM: Contrast-enhanced computed tomography and MRI provide complementary information in case of ROCM. The fol-

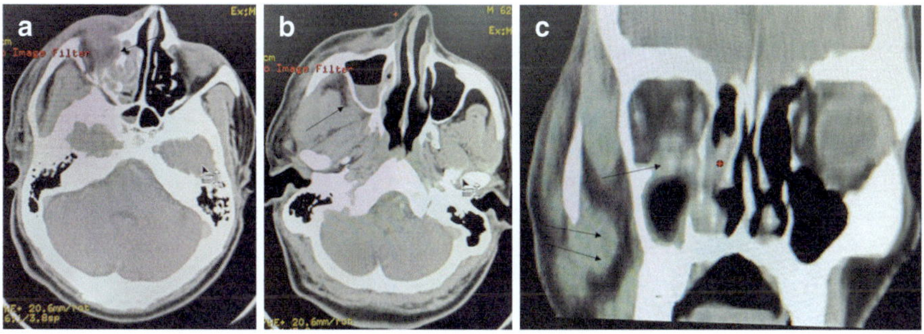

Fig. 10.5 Radiology in CAROM. (**a**) NCCT PNS revealing soft tissue in the anterior ethmoid with destruction of lamina papyracea (arrow). (**b**) Periantral fat streaking noted. (**c**) Orbital floor eroded with soft tissue tracking into the orbit and abutting inferior rectus muscle (single arrow). Accompanying inflammation seen over the premaxillary soft tissue (double arrow)

lowing radiological pointers are most often used to predict the possibility of ROCM [58]:

Presence of soft tissue in the paranasal sinuses with bone erosion.

Extrasinus spread of the disease without bone erosion signifies angio-invasiveness.

Extrasinus spread of the disease to involve the periantral fat is considered to be one of the earliest signs [59]

Fungal elements appear hypointense on T2-weighted MRI due to the presence of heavy metals. "Black turbinate" sign, where fungal elements in middle turbinate produce hypointensity of the middle turbinate, is considered one of the earliest signs of ROCM on MRI [60].

– To determine the extent of the disease:

Palatal involvement presents as bone erosion at the level of hard palate or through and through an oroantral fistula

The presence of extensive premaxillary soft tissue involvement with or without skin involvement may preclude a purely endoscopic approach.

The presence of soft tissue thickening in retroantral region and pterygomaxillary fissure necessitates an infratemporal fossa clearance.

Orbital involvement: The earliest signs of orbital invasion on radiology include soft tissue thickening at the level of the nasolacrimal duct, thickening of the medial rectus muscle, and retro-orbital fat stranding [58]. Progressive orbital involvement can be evinced by the presence of enlargement of all extraocular muscles, bone erosion at the level of lamina papyracea and inferior orbital wall, stretching and thickening of the optic nerve, presence of soft tissue at the orbital apex and superior orbital fissure, uveoscleral thickening (panophthalmitis), and tenting of the posterior pole of the globe (guitar pick sign) [58].

Intracranial involvement: Cavernous sinus involvement on MRI can be confirmed by the presence of altered signal intensity, enlargement of the superior ophthalmic vein, and bulky cavernous sinus. Intracranial involvement can range from erosion of cribriform plate, meningeal enhancement, signs of cerebritis, to abscess formation (peripheral ring-enhancing lesion). MRI should also be reviewed carefully to rule out any vascular complications like arteritis, carotid or basilar artery narrowing, or formation of a pseudoaneurysm [58].

10.4.5 Treatment

Management of CAROM should be performed by a multidisciplinary team involving otorhinolaryngologists, infectious disease experts, intensivists, prosthodontics, plastic and reconstructive surgeons, neurosurgeons, and neurologist. The best outcomes are obtained in patients diagnosed at Talmi stages I and II and those who undergo timely debridement and initiation of antifungal therapy. Therapeutic challenges unique to CAROM are as follows:

1. Timing of debridement: Surgical intervention for ROCM is time-sensitive. A delay of 6 days in surgical debridement can double the risk of 30-day mortality [49]. However, performing an extensive paranasal sinus debridement in a COVID-19-positive set-up poses safety risk to healthcare personnel involved and adds to perioperative morbidity for the patient. Knisely et al. have compared perioperative outcomes in COVID-19-positive patients undergoing emergency surgical intervention with non-COVID-19 patients undergoing similar procedures [61]. They reported 16.7% mortality in COVID-19-positive patients compared to 1.4% in COVID-19-negative patients, along with higher ICU admission rates (36.1 vs. 16.1%). Therefore, the decision regarding expedited surgery while the patient is concomitantly COVID-19-positive needs to be individualized, taking into consideration the severity of COVID-19 illness and the extent of ROCM [45]. Gupta et al. have proposed a decision-making algorithm for CAROM, considering the severity of COVID-19 illness and ROCM [45]. It was recommended that surgery might be deferred in low-severity ROCM for about 2 weeks to reduce COVID-19-associated perioperative morbidity. In case of high-severity ROCM, debridement should be expedited. If concomitant COVID-19 severity is mild or moderate, the patient needs to be taken up for surgery under the high-risk category. However, if COVID-19 severity falls in the severe category, debridement should be deferred till the intensivist considers the patient to be hemodynamically stable to undergo the procedure.
2. The extent of surgical resection: Surgical resection should aim to remove all necrotic and devitalized tissue and eliminate the nidus of fungus. However, this is impossible to achieve completely in cavernous sinus/intracranial involvement and sometimes inappropriate in case of peripheral or early orbital involvement due to the cosmetic and functional disability consequent to orbital debridement.

   The surgical approaches available for debridement of ROCM are endoscopic and open approaches. For patients requiring palatal resection, extensive involvement of premaxillary soft tissue and skin and those requiring orbital exenteration are not considered appropriate for purely endoscopic resection. Sublabial approach also offers excellent cosmetic results by avoiding facial incision in patients requiring only limited debridement.

3. Antifungal therapy: Intravenous liposomal amphotericin B is the first-line antifungal for ROCM. It should be administered at a dose of 3–6 mg/kg body weight/day. Initial high-dose treatment may limit the spread of infection, but high dosage treatment is often limited by toxicity (chills and rigors, allergic and anaphylactic reactions, dose-related nephrotoxicity). A cumulative dose of 3–5 g of amphotericin B is probably sufficient for patients with stage I/II disease wherein complete debridement is achieved. For intracranial disease, wherein complete debridement is almost never realistic, a cumulative dose of 8 g or maximum tolerable dose of amphotericin B is recommended [62].

   Oral posaconazole or isavuconazole is considered a step-down antifungal. Oral posaconazole is prescribed at a dose of 300 mg twice daily on the first day, followed by 300 mg once a day. Absorption is better when administered with a fatty meal. Serum drug level biological assays may be used to ascertain drug bioavailability.

10.5 Neuro-Otological Sequelae

1. Vertigo: Dizziness is one of the commonest neurological manifestations of COVID-19. There are anecdotal reports of vertigo persisting beyond the recovery of COVID-19 [63]. The possible causes for vertigo are vestibular neuronitis, benign paroxysmal positional vertigo, and posterior circulation stroke. Mechanisms of neuroinvasion that have been proposed include binding to ACE-2 receptors, hypercoagulopathy, hypoxia, and immune-mediated mechanisms [64, 65]. At present, there is little clarity about the outcome of COVID-19-associated dizziness. Vestibular rehabilitation measures have been shown to be of benefit [63].
2. Sensorineural hearing loss: Sudden sensorineural hearing loss (SSNHL) is defined as at least 30 dB hearing loss in three consecutive frequencies within 3 days. Post-viral SSNHL has been described with herpes virus and cytomegalovirus [66]. SSNHL in COVID-19 is now being recognized, especially following the recovery of the illness. SSNHL is frequently described with moderate and severe forms of the disease [67].

   Various theories surround the etiopathogenesis of SSNHL in COVID-19. The first hypothesis is direct damage to the epithelial cells of the organ of Corti, spiral ganglion, and the endothelial cells of stria vascularis. This is supported by the expression of ACE-2 receptors in these cells [68]. SARS-CoV-2-induced direct cochlear damage was revealed by Mustafa and colleagues, where COVID-19-infected patients were found to have a higher threshold in high frequencies and worsened threshold for transient evoked otoacoustic emission compared to normal individuals with no history of COVID-19 positivity [69]. The second plausible mechanism causing inner ear damage could arise from COVID-19-induced cytokine storm [70]. Hypercoagulopathy-induced ischemic damage to the inner ear has also been proposed as mechanism for inner ear damage due to COVID-19. Treatment of SSNHL occurring in the context of COVID-19 is not different from SSNHL due to other viral etiology. First-line management consists of oral corticosteroids. Intratympanic steroid is reserved for salvage in oral steroid-unresponsive cases.

3. Tinnitus: Due to the previously described mechanisms of inner ear damage, tinnitus and balance disorders may present in patients recovering from COVID-19 [71]. In a multicentric questionnaire-based study conducted in Italy on patients who were in the 30–60 days' interval from COVID-19 diagnosis, disequilibrium was reported in 18.4% of subjects and tinnitus in 23.2%, and 7.6% reported both disequilibrium and tinnitus [71]
4. Facial palsy: SARS-CoV-2 is a neurotropic virus owing to the expression of ACE-2 receptors in the brain and cranial and peripheral nerves [72]. There is a lack of evidence currently to validate the causal role of SARS-CoV-2 in the development of facial palsy in these patients.
5. Ototoxicity: Compounds containing quinine are known to cause inner ear damage [9]. Though there have been no reports of ototoxicity following hydroxychloroquine administration for COVID-19, it is important to be aware of this adverse effect [9]. Ototoxicity following hydroxychloroquine use can present long after discontinuation of the treatment and is known to be irreversible [9].

10.6 Upper Airway Dysfunction-Related Sequelae

1. Dysphonia: Incidence of dysphonia as a primary symptom of COVID-19 ranges from 26.8 to 43.7% [20, 73]. As per the study published by Cantarella et al., 15% of these patients have persistent dysphonia beyond 1 month following the diagnosis of COVID-19 [73]. Dysphonia in mild to moderate COVID-19 was significantly associated with smoking and upper airway symptoms like rhinitis and cough [20, 73]. To the contrary, the development of dysphonia in severe COVID-19 was associated with intubation granuloma, cord palsy, and use of nebulized glucocorticoid [74]. Underlying pathophysiology includes vocal cord strain from cough and rhinitis, recurrent laryngeal nerve damage from the virus, recurrent laryngeal nerve compression due to the endotracheal tube, and the "corditis" theory [74]. Direct virus-induced vocal cord inflammation or corditis is supported by the expression of ACE-2 receptors on vocal cord epithelium and the presence of isolated dysphonia in patients with no other upper airway inflammatory symptoms and no history of steroid use or endotracheal intubation [15, 74].
2. Tracheal stenosis: There have been anecdotal reports of tracheal stenosis developing secondary to prolonged intubation for severe COVID-19 [8]. This typically manifests as progressive shortness of breath and noisy breathing following a trial of extubation. Diagnosis can be confirmed on fiber-optic bronchoscopy,

X-ray soft tissue, and non-contrast computed tomography of the neck and chest. Bilateral cord palsy should be considered in the differential diagnosis. Management depends on the length of stenosis, the extent of airway compromise, and proximity to the subglottis. Tracheostomy is performed as an emergent measure to secure the airway. Subsequent treatment ranges from repeated endoscopic dilatation to resection of the stenosed segment and end to end anastomosis.

10.7 Sequelae Related to Upper Aerodigestive Tract-Lymphoreticular System

Kawasaki-like syndrome following COVID-19 infection has been described predominantly in the pediatric population and rarely in adults [75]. ENT manifestations include multiple cervical lymphadenopathies (most commonly jugulodigastric node) and oral mucosal lesions (strawberry tongue). Awareness among ENT practitioners is necessary since ENT manifestations often precede multisystem organ involvement [75].

10.8 Post-COVID-19 Thyroiditis

Subacute thyroiditis (SAT), also known as de Quervain's thyroiditis, has been described in association with post-COVID-19 sequelae. In a systematic review published by Rehman and colleagues, SAT symptoms appeared after an average of 25.2 ± 10.1 days from the diagnosis of COVID-19 [76]. SAT is a self-limiting condition progressing through three phases: hyperthyroid, hypothyroid, and euthyroid. It is associated with a rise in inflammatory serum markers (ESR and CRP). Management consists of nonsteroidal anti-inflammatory drugs and corticosteroids. Since SAT has previously been linked to viral illnesses like mumps, measles, rubella, coxsackievirus, and adenovirus, SAT in association with COVID-19 is also likely due to direct virus-induced damage or related to virus-induced inflammatory response [76, 77].

10.9 Take-Home Points

1. Post COVID 19 chemosensory dysfunction can be persistent in 7.2% of individuals.
2. Thorough ENT evaluation, the patient-reported structured questionnaires, paranasal sinus and brain imaging, and objective testing using quantitative olfactory testing complete the work-up for post-COVID-19 chemosensory dysfunction.
3. Evidence-based treatment recommendations are most robust for early initiation of olfactory training.
4. Topical steroid spray may be recommended along with olfactory training. Currently, there is a paucity of evidence favoring oral steroid administration.

5. Development of ROCM in the background of COVID-19 (CAROM) can be linked to uncontrolled hyperglycemia, steroid administration, COVID-19-induced iron overload state, immunosuppression arising from IL-6 antagonist use, and decrease in phagocyte activity and hypercoagulability.
6. In patients with a high index of suspicion toward CAROM, the diagnosis can be rendered following 10% KOH examination of the tissue and imaging of the paranasal sinus and brain.
7. Treatment of CAROM should include timely initiation of amphotericin B and timely surgical debridement. Oral posaconazole is used as a step-down antifungal.
8. Involvement of orbit, cavernous sinus, and intracranial extension ported a poor outcome with high mortality rates.

References

1. El-Anwar MW, Elzayat S, Fouad YA. ENT manifestation in COVID-19 patients. Auris Nasus Larynx [Internet] 2020 Jun 15 [cited 2020 Aug 24]; Available from https://www.ncbi.nlm.nih.gov/pmc/articles/PMC7294298/
2. Panda S, Mohamed A, Sikka K, Kanodia A, Sakthivel P, Thakar A, et al. Otolaryngologic manifestation and long-term outcome in mild COVID-19: experience from a tertiary care Centre in India. Indian J Otolaryngol Head Neck Surg. 2020;73(1):1–6.
3. Krajewska J, Krajewski W, Zub K, Zatoński T. COVID-19 in otolaryngologist practice: a review of current knowledge. Eur Arch Otorhinolaryngol. 2020;277(7):1885–97.
4. Lechner M, Liu J, Counsell N, Ta NH, Rocke J, Anmolsingh R, et al. Course of symptoms for loss of sense of smell and taste over time in one thousand forty-one healthcare workers during the Covid-19 pandemic: our experience. Clin Otolaryngol. 2021;46(2):451–7.
5. Paderno A, Mattavelli D, Rampinelli V, Grammatica A, Raffetti E, Tomasoni M, et al. Olfactory and gustatory outcomes in COVID-19: a prospective evaluation in nonhospitalized subjects. Otolaryngol Head Neck Surg. 2020 Dec;163(6):1144–9.
6. National Comprehensive Guidelines for Management of Post Covid Sequelae.pdf [Internet]. [cited 2021 Dec 9]. Available from https://www.mohfw.gov.in/pdf/NationalComprehensiveGuidelinesforManagementofPostCovidSequelae.pdf
7. Hussain S, Baxi H, Riad A, Klugarová J, Pokorná A, Slezáková S, et al. COVID-19-associated Mucormycosis (CAM): an updated evidence mapping. Int J Environ Res Public Health. 2021;18(19):10340.
8. Giordano D, Botti C, Castellucci A, Piro R, Ghidini A. Tracheal stenosis after tracheotomy for COVID-19. Ear Nose Throat J. 2021:1455613211045539.
9. De Luca P, Scarpa A, De Bonis E, Cavaliere M, Viola P, Gioacchini FM, et al. Chloroquine and hydroxychloroquine ototoxicity; potential implications for SARS-CoV-2 treatment. A brief review of the literature. Am J Otolaryngol. 2021;42(5):102640.
10. van Kempen M, Bachert C, Van Cauwenberge P. An update on the pathophysiology of rhinovirus upper respiratory tract infections. Rhinology. 1999;37(3):97–103.
11. Suzuki M, Saito K, Min W-P, Vladau C, Toida K, Itoh H, et al. Identification of viruses in patients with postviral olfactory dysfunction. Laryngoscope. 2007;117(2):272–7.
12. Hummel T, Whitcroft KL, Andrews P, Altundag A, Cinghi C, Costanzo RM, et al. Position paper on olfactory dysfunction. Rhinology. 2016;56(1):1–30.
13. Damm M, Temmel A, Welge-Lüssen A, Eckel HE, Kreft M-P, Klussmann JP, et al. [Olfactory dysfunctions. Epidemiology and therapy in Germany, Austria and Switzerland]. HNO 2004 ;52(2):112–120.

14. Temmel AFP, Quint C, Schickinger-Fischer B, Klimek L, Stoller E, Hummel T. Characteristics of olfactory disorders in relation to major causes of olfactory loss. Arch Otolaryngol Neck Surg. 2002;128(6):635–41.
15. Lechien JR, Chiesa-Estomba CM, De Siati DR, Horoi M, Le Bon SD, Rodriguez A, et al. Olfactory and gustatory dysfunctions as a clinical presentation of mild-to-moderate forms of the coronavirus disease (COVID-19): a multicenter European study. Eur Arch Otorhinolaryngol. 2020;277(8):2251–61.
16. von Bartheld CS, Hagen MM, Butowt R. Prevalence of chemosensory dysfunction in COVID-19 patients: a systematic review and meta-analysis reveals significant ethnic differences. ACS Chem Neurosci. 2020;11(19):2944–61.
17. Kaye R, Chang CWD, Kazahaya K, Brereton J, Denneny JC. COVID-19 anosmia reporting tool: initial findings. Otolaryngol Head Neck Surg. 2020;163(1):132–4.
18. Addison AB, Wong B, Ahmed T, Macchi A, Konstantinidis I, Huart C, et al. Clinical Olfactory Working Group consensus statement on the treatment of post-infectious olfactory dysfunction. J Allergy Clin Immunol. 2021;147(5):1704–19.
19. Vaira LA, Hopkins C, Petrocelli M, Lechien JR, Chiesa-Estomba CM, Salzano G, et al. Smell and taste recovery in coronavirus disease 2019 patients: a 60-day objective and prospective study. J Laryngol Otol. 2020;134(8):703–9.
20. Lechien JR, Chiesa-Estomba CM, Vaira LA, Saussez S, Hans S. COVID-19 reinfection and second episodes of olfactory and gustatory dysfunctions: report of first cases. Ear Nose Throat J. 2020:145561320970105.
21. Liu DT, Sabha M, Damm M, Philpott C, Oleszkiewicz A, Hähner A, et al. Parosmia is associated with relevant olfactory recovery after olfactory training. Laryngoscope. 2021;131(3):618–23.
22. Rombaux P, Huart C, Deggouj N, Duprez T, Hummel T. Prognostic value of olfactory bulb volume measurement for recovery in post-infectious and posttraumatic olfactory loss. Otolaryngol Head Neck Surg. 2012 Dec;147(6):1136–41.
23. Parma V, Ohla K, Veldhuizen MG, Niv MY, Kelly CE, Bakke AJ, et al. More than smell-COVID-19 is associated with severe impairment of smell, taste, and chemesthesis. Chem Senses. 2020;45(7):609–22.
24. Yamagishi M, Fujiwara M, Nakamura H. Olfactory mucosal findings and clinical course in patients with olfactory disorders following upper respiratory viral infection. Rhinology. 1994;32(3):113–8.
25. Jafek BW, Murrow B, Michaels R, Restrepo D, Linschoten M. Biopsies of human olfactory epithelium. Chem Senses. 2002;27(7):623–8.
26. Bryche B, St Albin A, Murri S, Lacôte S, Pulido C, ArGouilh M, et al. Massive transient damage of the olfactory epithelium associated with infection of sustentacular cells by SARS-CoV-2 in golden Syrian hamsters. Brain Behav Immun. 2020;89:579–86.
27. Bilinska K, Jakubowska P, Von Bartheld CS, Butowt R. Expression of the SARS-CoV-2 entry proteins, ACE2 and TMPRSS2, in cells of the olfactory epithelium: identification of cell types and trends with age. ACS Chem Neurosci. 2020;11(11):1555–62.
28. Yıldız E, Balcı A, Selendili O, Kuzu S. Olfactory cleft opacification in COVID-19 related smell loss: CT findings and correlation with objective testing. Ear Nose Throat J. 2021:1455613211011285.
29. Webster KE, O'Byrne L, MacKeith S, Philpott C, Hopkins C, Burton MJ. Interventions for the prevention of persistent post-COVID-19 olfactory dysfunction. Cochrane Database Syst Rev. 2021,7.CD013877.
30. Abdelalim AA, Mohamady AA, Elsayed RA, Elawady MA, Ghallab AF. Corticosteroid nasal spray for recovery of smell sensation in COVID-19 patients: a randomized controlled trial. Am J Otolaryngol. 2021;42(2):102884.
31. Pekala K, Chandra RK, Turner JH. Efficacy of olfactory training in patients with olfactory loss: a systematic review and meta-analysis. Int Forum Allergy Rhinol. 2016;6(3):299–307.
32. Sorokowska A, Drechsler E, Karwowski M, Hummel T. Effects of olfactory training: a meta-analysis. Rhinology. 2017;55(1):17–26.

33. Fukazawa K. A local steroid injection method for olfactory loss due to upper respiratory infection. Chem Senses. 2005;30(Suppl1):i212–3.
34. Yuan F, Huang T, Wei Y, Wu D. Steroids and olfactory training for postviral olfactory dysfunction: a systematic review. Front Neurosci. 2021;15:708510.
35. Mori E, Merkonidis C, Cuevas M, Gudziol V, Matsuwaki Y, Hummel T. The administration of nasal drops in the "Kaiteki" position allows for delivery of the drug to the olfactory cleft: a pilot study in healthy subjects. Eur Arch Otorhinolaryngol. 2016 Apr;273(4):939–43.
36. İşlek A, Balcı MK. Phantosmia with COVID-19 related olfactory dysfunction: report of nine case. Indian J Otolaryngol Head Neck Surg. 2021:1–3.
37. Eucker J, Sezer O, Graf B, Possinger K. Mucormycoses. Mycoses. 2001;44(7–8):253–60.
38. Prakash H, Chakrabarti A. Epidemiology of mucormycosis in India. Microorganisms. 2021;9(3):523.
39. Sugar AM. Mucormycosis. Clin Infect Dis. 1992;14(Suppl1):S126–9.
40. Smith HW, Kirchner JA. Cerebral mucormycosis; a report of three cases. AMA Arch Otolaryngol. 1958 Dec;68(6):715–26.
41. Singh AK, Singh R, Joshi SR, Misra A. Mucormycosis in COVID-19: a systematic review of cases reported worldwide and in India. Diabetes Metab Syndr. 2021;15(4):102146.
42. Talmi YP, Goldschmied-Reouven A, Bakon M, Barshack I, Wolf M, Horowitz Z, et al. Rhino-orbital and rhino-orbito-cerebral mucormycosis. Otolaryngol Head Neck Surg. 2002 Jul;127(1):22–31.
43. Mucormycosis [Internet]. [cited 2021 Dec 29]. Available from https://www.who.int/india/emergencies/coronavirus-disease-(covid-19)/mucormycosis
44. Raut A, Huy NT. Rising incidence of mucormycosis in patients with COVID-19: another challenge for India amidst the second wave? Lancet Respir Med. 2021;9(8):e77.
45. Gupta NK, Kapre M, Gupta H, Vaidya GK, Jani S, Meshram S, et al. Risk based decision algorithms for management of COVID-19 associated rhino-orbital mucormycosis. Indian J Otolaryngol Head Neck Surg. 2021;30:1–8.
46. Garg R, Bharangar S, Gupta S, Bhardwaj S. Post Covid-19 infection presenting as rhino-orbital mycosis. Indian J Otolaryngol Head Neck Surg. 2021;14:1–8.
47. Thakar A, Lal D. "Black fungus": a perspective on the coronavirus disease 2019 (COVID-19)-associated rhino-orbital mucormycosis epidemic in India. Int Forum Allergy Rhinol. 2021;11(8):1278–9.
48. Singh A, Sikka K, Goel G, Kanodia A, Chandran A, Konkimalla A, et al. COVID associated rhino-orbito-cerebral mucormycosis in Delhi (CAROM)—demographics and risk factors in a single centre consecutive cohort of 200 patients. Natl Med J India. 2022;15:3505–14.
49. Sen M, Lahane S, Lahane TP, Parekh R, Honavar SG. Mucor in a viral land: a tale of two pathogens. Indian J Ophthalmol. 2021;69(2):244–52.
50. Kothandaraman N, Rengaraj A, Xue B, Yew WS, Velan SS, Karnani N, et al. COVID-19 endocrinopathy with hindsight from SARS. Am J Physiol Endocrinol Metab. 2021;320(1):E139–50.
51. Baldin C, Ibrahim AS. Molecular mechanisms of mucormycosis—the bitter and the sweet. PLoS Pathog. 2017;13(8):e1006408.
52. Chen G, Wu D, Guo W, Cao Y, Huang D, Wang H, et al. Clinical and immunological features of severe and moderate coronavirus disease 2019. J Clin Invest. 2020;130(5):2620–9.
53. Ibrahim TF, Jahromi BR, Miettinen J, Raj R, Andrade-Barazarte H, Goehre F, et al. Long-term causes of death and excess mortality after carotid artery ligation. World Neurosurg. 2016;90:116–22.
54. Coutinho AE, Chapman KE. The anti-inflammatory and immunosuppressive effects of glucocorticoids, recent developments and mechanistic insights. Mol Cell Endocrinol. 2011;335(1):2–13.
55. National Institutes of Health. COVID-19 treatments and vaccines [Internet]. NIH COVID-19 Research. [cited 2021 Dec 29]. Available from https://covid19.nih.gov/treatments-and-vaccines
56. Muthu V, et al. Is there an association between zinc and COVID-19-associated mucormycosis? Results of an experimental and clinical study. Mycoses. 2021:1291–7.

57. Bala K, Chander J, Handa U, Punia RS, Attri AK. A prospective study of mucormycosis in North India: experience from a tertiary care hospital. Med Mycol. 2015;53(3):248–57.
58. Manchanda S, Semalti K, Bhalla AS, Thakar A, Sikka K, Verma H. Revisiting rhino-orbito-cerebral acute invasive fungal sinusitis in the era of COVID-19: pictorial review. Emerg Radiol. 2021;28(6):1063–72.
59. Middlebrooks EH, Frost CJ, De Jesus RO, Massini TC, Schmalfuss IM, Mancuso AA. Acute invasive fungal rhinosinusitis: a comprehensive update of CT findings and design of an effective diagnostic imaging model. AJNR Am J Neuroradiol. 2015;36(8):1529–35.
60. Honavar SG. Code Mucor: guidelines for the diagnosis, staging and management of rhino-orbito-cerebral mucormycosis in the setting of COVID-19. Indian J Ophthalmol. 2021;69(6):1361–5.
61. Knisely A, Zhou ZN, Wu J, Huang Y, Holcomb K, Melamed A, et al. Perioperative morbidity and mortality of patients with COVID-19 who undergo urgent and emergent surgical procedures. Ann Surg. 2021;273(1):34–40.
62. Vaid N, Mishra P, Gokhale N, Vaid S, Vaze V, Kothadiya A, et al. A proposed grading system and experience of COVID-19 associated rhino orbito cerebral mucormycosis from an Indian tertiary care center. Indian J Otolaryngol Head Neck Surg. 2021;15:1–8.
63. Saniasiaya J, Kulasegarah J. Dizziness and COVID-19. Ear Nose Throat J. 2020;100(1):29–30. https://doi.org/10.1177/0145561320959573.
64. Baig AM, Khaleeq A, Ali U, Syeda H. Evidence of the COVID-19 virus targeting the CNS: tissue distribution, host–virus interaction, and proposed neurotropic mechanisms. ACS Chem Neurosci. 2020;11(7):995.
65. Wu Y, Xu X, Chen Z, Duan J, Hashimoto K, Yang L, et al. Nervous system involvement after infection with COVID-19 and other coronaviruses. Brain Behav Immun. 2020;1(87):18–22.
66. Cohen BE, Durstenfeld A, Roehm PC. Viral causes of hearing loss: a review for hearing health professionals. Trends Hear. 2014;22(18):2331216514541361.
67. Koumpa FS, Forde CT, Manjaly JG. Sudden irreversible hearing loss post COVID-19. BMJ Case Rep. 2020;13(11):e238419.
68. Uranaka T, Kashio A, Ueha R, Sato T, Bing H, Ying G, et al. Expression of ACE2, TMPRSS2, and furin in mouse ear tissue, and the implications for SARS-CoV-2 infection. Laryngoscope. 2021;131(6):E2013–7.
69. Mustafa MWM. Audiological profile of asymptomatic Covid-19 PCR-positive cases. Am J Otolaryngol. 2020;41(3):102483.
70. Vallamkondu J, John A, Wani WY, Ramadevi SP, Jella KK, Reddy PH, et al. SARS-CoV-2 pathophysiology and assessment of coronaviruses in CNS diseases with a focus on therapeutic targets. Biochim Biophys Acta Mol Basis Dis. 2020;1866(10):165889.
71. Viola P, Ralli M, Pisani D, Malanga D, Sculco D, Messina L, et al. Tinnitus and equilibrium disorders in COVID-19 patients: preliminary results. Eur Arch Otorhinolaryngol. 2021;278(10):3725–30.
72. Ozer F, Alkan O. Simultaneous sudden hearing loss and peripheral facial paralysis in a patient with Covid-19. Ear Nose Throat J. 2021;5:1455613211028094.
73. Cantarella G, Aldè M, Consonni D, Zuccotti G, Berardino FD, Barozzi S, et al. Prevalence of dysphonia in non hospitalized patients with COVID-19 in Lombardy, the Italian epicenter of the pandemic. J Voice [Internet] 2021 Mar 14 [cited 2021 Dec 30].
74. Leis-Coñño C, Arriero-Sánchez P, González-Herranz R, Arenas-Brítez Ó, Hernández-García E, Plaza G. Persistent Dysphonia in Hospitalized COVID-19 Patients. J Voice [Internet]. 2021 Jul 24 [cited 2021 Dec 30]; Available from https://www.ncbi.nlm.nih.gov/pmc/articles/PMC8302831/
75. Lechien JR, Hervochon R, Hans S. Post-COVID-19 Kawasaki-like syndrome. Ear Nose Throat J. 2021;26:1455613211006011.
76. Aemaz Ur Rehman M, Farooq H, Ali MM, Ebaad Ur Rehman M, Dar QA, Hussain A. The Association of Subacute Thyroiditis with COVID-19: a systematic review. SN Compr Clin Med. 2021,29:1–13.
77. Desailloud R, Hober D. Viruses and thyroiditis: an update. Virol J. 2009;12(6):5.

Rheumatological Complications Following COVID-19

11

Rudra Prosad Goswami and Uma Kumar

With the prolongation of the pandemic, several observational and epidemiologic studies have started to report on persistent symptoms after resolution of acute infection of Covid-19 beyond 3 months [1]. The incidence of such manifestations has been reported to be as high as 30% [2]. Several of these manifestations are musculoskeletal, and rarely the patients develop de novo systemic autoimmune diseases fulfilling guideline-based classification criteria. Several mechanisms of such de novo autoimmunity have been proposed which include molecular mimicry, bystander effect, persistent immune activation and NETosis among others [2]. In this review we summarize the various musculoskeletal and autoimmune diseases that develop after resolution of Covid-19 infection.

11.1 Musculoskeletal Manifestations

Infections are known triggers of autoimmunity and rheumatic diseases are no exception. The most classic example would be post-urethritis or post-diarrhoeal reactive arthritis. Viral infections are known triggers of multiple autoimmune diseases like systemic lupus erythematosus (SLE) or Sjögren's syndrome among others.

Post-Covid-19 musculoskeletal problems range from mild to moderate arthralgia, reactive arthritis to full-blown classifiable arthritis syndromes like rheumatoid arthritis [2].

R. P. Goswami · U. Kumar (✉)
Department of Rheumatology, AIIMS, New Delhi, India

A. Mohan, S. Mittal (eds.), *Post COVID-19 Complications and Management*,
https://doi.org/10.1007/978-981-19-4407-9_11

11.1.1 Arthralgia

Arthralgia is the commonest musculoskeletal manifestation of long Covid syndrome and has been reported widely and repeatedly [2, 3]. A recent systematic review and meta-analysis, still in pre-print form, reported that one in every five patients with long Covid complains of arthralgia [4].

11.1.2 Reactive Arthritis

Several mechanisms of reactive arthritis following viral infections have been proposed including molecular mimicry among others. SARS-CoV-2 proteins have displayed match with the human proteins on a comparative peptidome analysis comprising of 37 viral proteins [5]. Mimicking epitopes may be present in intra-articular locations and perhaps on the synovial lining resulting in acute inflammation. Two recent systematic searches of the PubMed and Scopus platform identified 22 published cases of post-Covid-19 reactive arthritis published between January 2020 and July 2021 [6, 7]. Average gap between onset of Covid-19 symptoms and acute arthritis was 25 days (range 7–90 days). Knees and ankles were the commonly inflamed joints; however tenosynovitis, sacroiliitis, and small joints were also involved in a smaller number of cases. HLA-B27 was positive in four out of seven cases tested. Majority were treated with oral nonsteroidal agents with or without intra-articular corticosteroids, and all recovered with no residual stigmata of joint disease in up to 6 months of follow-up. This rather low prevalence may represent publication bias. On the other hand, the diagnosis of reactive arthritis is essentially that of an exclusion after a long and tedious list of possibilities which includes but is not confined to crystal disease, early systemic arthritis, early connective tissue disease and an apparently inexhaustible panel of viral and bacterial markers. Interestingly five cases were tested for RT-PCR of SARS-CoV-2 in the aspirated synovial fluid which were negative [7]. Clinically the lesson that these published cases tell us is that post-Covid-19 reactive arthritis behaves in a similar fashion as that of the garden-variety post-bacterial reactive arthritis, and judiciously limited treatment suffices.

11.1.3 Rheumatoid Arthritis (RA)

There are a few published reports of development of RA following Covid-19 infection. A Dutch cohort described five patients with inflammatory arthritis presenting on an average of 6.6 weeks after moderately severe Covid-19 infection four of whom fulfilled the American College of Rheumatology 2010 criteria [8]. The authors diagnosed only three of them as clinical RA, two had strong positive anticyclic citrullinated peptide antibody (ACPA) and one had weak positive ACPA. In detailed phenotype of these new-onset ACPAs, the authors observed that the percentage of V-domain glycosylation was increased similar to regular RA patients.

There are also ten other reported cases of seropositive and seronegative RA all of whom developed the disease 4–6 weeks after Covid-19 infection [2, 9–11]. Treatment was in usual lines as that of regular RA. However, causation is difficult to establish as serology status before the infection is hardly reported in any case.

11.1.4 Myositis

Muscle involvement after Covid-19 infection is varied and ranges from non-specific myalgia, asymptomatic mild to moderate rise in creatine kinase (CK) to full-blown inflammatory myositis to rhabdomyolysis [2, 12]. In one study myalgia was present in early half of the patients and raised CK was reported in nearly one third of all the patients [13]. Frank myositis is observed, though rarely, after Covid-19 infection. Phenotypically the reported cases are similar to other postinfectious myositis as seen after respiratory viral infections or dengue viral infection.

Patients present with myalgia and often low-grade fever followed by progressive symmetric proximal weakness and elevated CK. Muscle biopsy is non-specific and shows focal lymphocytic infiltrates and it is unusual to show biopsy hallmarks of dermatomyositis. Autoantibodies are distinct by their absence, though low-titre antinuclear antibodies (ANA) may be positive. Reported patients have received a variety of treatments like glucocorticoids, hydroxychloroquine and methotrexate usually with a good response [14–16]. There are only a few reports of frank dermatomyositis with autoantibodies like anti-Mi2 ($n = 1$), anti-MDA5 ($n = 1$), anti-SAE1 ($n = 2$) or antinuclear autoantibodies ($n = 1$) preceded by Covid-19 [17]. In these cases causation is always difficult but pathogenic association could be postulated. There are some evidences that Covid-19 could trigger the MDA-5 or RIG-like innate immunity pathogen sensing pathways that may lead to muscle inflammation [18]. Rebendenne et al. showed human airway epithelial cells elicit a strong interferon response to Covid-19 infection and that the melanoma differentiation-associated gene (MDA) 5 is its main biological sensor in the human pulmonary parenchyma. The link between Covid-19 infection and muscle damage or inflammation was suggested by an autopsy study where the authors included patients who died from Covid-19 ($n = 43$) or other critical illnesses ($n = 11$) and inflammation of skeletal muscle was assessed by quantitative estimates of inflammatory cell infiltrates and MHC-I and MHC-II. Interestingly samples from patients with Covid-19 showed consistently higher pathology score, inflammation scores and higher expression of MHCs [19]. However this cannot be taken as a conclusive evidence as myositis as these results could be alternately interpreted as scattered or spotty MHC-I expression and as there was an absence of classic defining muscle histo-/immunopathology [20]. There are quite a few other important and interesting focal myositis syndromes described after Covid-19 infection like the paraspinal myositis syndrome [21], orbital myositis syndrome [22], myofascial compartment syndrome [23], cachexia [24] and axonal denervation and residual muscle degeneration among others [25].

11.2 Vasculitis/Thrombosis

Vasculitis and thrombosis are part of pathogenesis of Covid-19. Given that endothelial cell inflammation, apoptosis and finally endothelial dysfunction occur in patients with Covid-19 and a major viral entry site for viruses is heparan sulphate moieties on the endothelial cells, syndromes of vascular insufficiency manifested either as thrombosis characteristic of antiphospholipid syndrome or multiorgan manifestations like primary systemic vasculitis is within the expected spectrum of post-Covid-19 syndromes [26]. Several different manifestations of vasculitis secondary of Covid-19 have been reported, ranging from chilblains in the toes (Covid toe) [27], cutaneous leucocytoclastic vasculitis [28], acute limb ischaemia [29], retinal artery ischaemia [30], mesenteric vasculitis [31], diffuse alveolar haemorrhage [32], cerebral vasculitis with brainstem involvement [33] to primary systemic vasculitis with anti-neutrophil cytoplasmic antibody (ANCA) positivity [26]. Majority of these manifestations occur during the active infection, and some authors have found positive RT-PCR against Covid-19 from aspirates of accessible lesions [34]. However there are other reports of vasculitis developing 4–6 weeks after resolution of active infection suggesting immunological mechanisms and breakdown of tolerance.

The current authors have seen two cases of post-Covid-19 ANCA vasculitis. One was a 25-year-old man who developed severe anterior uveitis with scleromalacia 6 weeks after recovering from a mild Covid-19 infection. The second was a 55-year-old man who developed pulmonary cavitation and crescentic glomerulonephritis 4 weeks after recovering from mild to moderate Covid-19 infection. Both of them were positive for c-ANCA and anti-PR3 antibodies with high titre. Both had these vasculitic symptoms first time in their life. They were treated as per EUVAS protocol with cyclophosphamide followed by rituximab and only rituximab, respectively, with good outcome. There are several other reported cases of ANCA-associated vasculitis following Covid-19 infection [35, 36]. The presentation mimicked that of idiopathic ANCA-associated vasculitis (AAV) with a predominance of crescent glomerulonephritis. However, there was a predominance of anti-PR3 antibody, similar to our observation, suggesting further evidence for infectious antigen stimulation.

During the 2020 Covid-19 peaks, several reports emerged from western Europe highlighting an increased frequency of giant cell arteritis (GCA) [37, 38]. One report also highlighted possible increased ophthalmic complications of GCA during the pandemic [38]. This was further explored by a French group which systematically analysed their new and previously diagnosed GCA cases and observed that their centre experienced higher frequency of GCA during the pandemic albeit with an increased otorhinolaryngological manifestations rather than ophthalmic complications [39]. They also performed RT-PCR of the available temporal artery biopsy samples which were negative suggesting no role of active Covid-19 infection causing this symptomatology. On the other hand, majority of their patients were negative for serology against Covid-19, which casts doubt on possible immunological modulation by previous exposure to Covid-19. It is, however, useful to remember that both these diseases share common phenotypes like headache, fatigue and elevated inflammatory markers with significant differences like jaw claudication and thrombocytosis which are almost exclusively seen in GCA [40].

Antiphospholipid antibodies (aPL) have been noted in patients with infections and may predispose an infected individual to a prothrombotic state and present another potential mechanism of clinical manifestation through vascular insufficiency, ischaemia and necrosis. There have been several studies which showed a disproportionately elevated positivity rate of antiphospholipid antibodies among patients with Covid-19. For example, Harzallah et al. reported in 56 patients positive lupus anticoagulant in 25 and positive anti-beta-2 glycoprotein I (GPI) or anticardiolipin (ACL) in 5 patients [41]. Another study by Fan et al. reported lupus anticoagulant to be present in 50% of patients with severe disease requiring ICU admission and low-titre anti-ACL positivity [42]. Several issues have been raised against these reports and several other reports which highlight assay characteristics and reporting guidelines. Some of the objections raised are as follows: possible false positive lupus anticoagulant test due to ongoing anticoagulation; interaction of high CRP with the lupus anticoagulant-specific aPTT test; low-titre positivity of anti-ACL or anti-beta-2 GPI antibodies not fulfilling classification criteria; lack of reporting on persistent positivity; lack of reporting on anti-beta-2 GPI DI antibodies; and variability of assay and ELISA techniques [43, 44]. A few case reports have emerged that highlight persistent antiphospholipid antibodies even after 1 year after resolution of the active infection. Two studies reported on repeated antiphospholipid antibodies, in which one study showed persistent positivity in only one out of ten patients after 1 month and another reported three patients with persistent aPL positivity, after almost 3 months [45]. There are a few reports of clinical association of these antibodies. Two cases were reported with postural orthostatic tachycardia syndrome (POTS) persistent for almost 1 year after resolution of active infection, one with low-titre anti-beta-2 glycoprotein I IgM antibody and another with high-titre anti-beta-2-glycoprotein 1 IgM and anti-phosphatidylethanolamine IgM antibodies [45, 46]. Another case was reported with persistent IgG ACL antibody comprising of bizarre neurological constellations like headache, memory problems and chest pain without any clinical signs of thrombosis [47]. Perhaps the most disconcerting is the report of three cases with myocardial infarction and ventricular fibrillation occuring 3–6 months after Covid-19, among which one had weakly positive lupus anticoagulant [48].

11.3 Connective Tissue Disease

Covid-19 shares several features with systemic lupus erythematosus (SLE)-related features, like cytopenia, arthralgias, serositis, cutaneous lesions like chilblains and antibodies like antinuclear antibodies and antiphospholipid antibodies [49]. Few cases have been reported with full-blown lupus developing from 13 days to 1 month after onset of the Covid-19-related illness [50]. All had severe manifestations of lupus like macrophage activation syndrome, cardiac tamponade, acute kidney injury, polyserositis, etc., had multiple autoantibodies and required several immunosuppressives for adequate disease control. Though at face value these patients would fulfil the classification criteria for SLE, it is unclear whether they share the chronicity associated with typical idiopathic SLE or whether these are a transient severe immunological manifestation of Covid-19 itself, as they share clinical, immunological and therapeutic parameters with each other. There are a few cases of SLE developing after resolution of Covid-19 infection [51–54]. Clinical manifestations were typical of lupus characterized by skin rashes, arthralgia and proteinuria along with positive ANA and hypocomplementemia. While one case occurred during the tail end of Covid-19 infection and resulted in death of the patient, the other two cases presented 2 months after resolution of Covid-19. Various viral aetiologies as predisposing or triggering events have been postulated time and again in the long history towards our current and yet partial understanding of the disease complex named lupus that includes but is certainly not confined to the likes of the Epstein-Barr virus, cytomegalovirus, parvovirus B19 and retroviruses [55]. Maybe Covid-19 is another addendum to this list. None of these reports excluded other viral aetiologies, and even while present, the causal association is tenuous at most in the majority of cases.

11.4 Covid-19 Among Patients with Rheumatic Diseases

Patients with systemic autoimmune diseases suffer from dysfunction of the immune system that restricts their ability to mount an adequate response to an infectious trigger, and the drugs that are used to treat their diseases are invariably immunosuppressants which also increase risk of infection and serious adverse effects. This increases a theoretical risk of increased incidence of Covid-19 and possibly poorer outcome. An initial report from the COVID-19 Global Rheumatology Alliance international physician registry reported that patients on higher glucocorticoid doses show increase probability of hospitalization and those on anti-TNF drugs have lower probability [56], and even an increased risk of death was reported by another group of authors [57]. A recent meta-analysis dealt with this issue analysing 62 observational studies with a total of 319,025 patients with systemic autoimmune and inflammatory diseases (SAIIRD). The authors reported that the risk of Covid-19 in SAIIRD was significantly higher than controls (odds ratio: 2.19) and glucocorticoids were significantly associated with this risk. Interestingly, the authors reported that patients on biological or targeted synthetic disease-modifying agent monotherapy were at a lower risk of severe Covid-19 infection [58].

11.5 Conclusions

Post-Covid-19 or long Covid syndrome is an immunological phenomenon that burdens Covid-19 survivors. The immune aberration caused by Covid-19 infection shares several immunological traits associated with systemic autoimmune diseases, like plasmacytoid dendritic cell upregulation and interferon pathway activation.

However, apart from non-specific arthralgia, other well-defined systemic diseases like vasculitis, myositis, rheumatoid arthritis or systemic lupus are uncommon. Given the huge number of global cases of Covid-19 and a high burden of post-Covid-19 or long Covid syndrome, these cases, at least statistically would not fulfil any criteria of causation. But the issue with publication bias always confounds interpretation of such measures. Whatever be the case, the de novo cases behave almost in an identical manner as with their idiopathic counterparts, and all it requires from the clinician is wise observation and active management.

References

1. Garrigues E, Janvier P, Kherabi Y, et al. Post-discharge persistent symptoms and health-related quality of life after hospitalization for COVID-19. J Infect. 2020;81:e4–6.
2. Sapkota HR, Nune A. Long COVID from rheumatology perspective—a narrative review. Clin Rheumatol. 2021;41(2):337–48. https://doi.org/10.1007/s10067-021-06001-1.
3. Petersen MS, Kristiansen MF, Hanusson KD, Danielsen ME, Steig BÁ, Gaini S, Strøm M, Weihe P. Long COVID in the Faroe Islands—a longitudinal study among non-hospitalized patients. Clin Infect Dis. 2020;73(11):e4058–63.
4. Lopez-Leon S, Wegman-Ostrosky T, Perelman C, Sepulveda R, Rebolledo PA, Cuapio A, Villapol S. More than 50 long-term effects of COVID-19: a systematic review and meta-analysis. MedRxiv. 2021; https://doi.org/10.1101/2021.01.27.21250617.
5. Lyons-Weiler J. Pathogenic priming likely contributes to serious and critical illness and mortality in COVID-19 via autoimmunity. J Transl Autoimmun. 2020;3:100051.
6. Gasparotto M, Framba V, Piovella C, Doria A, Iaccarino L. Post-COVID-19 arthritis: a case report and literature review. Clin Rheumatol. 2021;40:3357–62.
7. Kocyigit BF, Akyol A. Reactive arthritis after COVID-19: a case-based review. Rheumatol Int. 2021;41:2031–9.
8. Derksen VFAM, Kissel T, Lamers-Karnebeek FBG, van der Bijl AE, Venhuizen AC, Huizinga TWJ, Toes REM, Roukens AHE, van der Woude D. Onset of rheumatoid arthritis after COVID-19: coincidence or connected? Ann Rheum Dis. 2021;80(8):1096–8. https://doi.org/10.1136/annrheumdis-2021-219859.
9. Tamborrini G, Micheroli R. [CME rheumatology 23/answers: rheumatoid arthritis following COVID-19/SARS-CoV-2 infection]. Praxis. 2021;110:375–6.
10. Perrot L, Hemon M, Busnel J-M, Muis-Pistor O, Picard C, Zandotti C, Pham T, Roudier J, Desplat-Jego S, Balandraud N. First flare of ACPA-positive rheumatoid arthritis after SARS-CoV-2 infection. Lancet Rheumatol. 2021;3:e6–8.
11. Ben-Chetrit E, Ben-Chetrit E. Palindromic rheumatism following COVID-19 infection evolved to rheumatoid arthritis after COVID-19 reinfection. Clin Exp Rheumatol. 2021;39:1410–2.
12. Chan KH, Farouji I, Abu Hanoud A, Slim J. Weakness and elevated creatinine kinase as the initial presentation of coronavirus disease 2019 (COVID-19). Am J Emerg Med. 2020;38:1548.e1–3.
13. Batur EB, Korez MK, Gezer IA, Levendoglu F, Ural O. Musculoskeletal symptoms and relationship with laboratory findings in patients with COVID-19. Int J Clin Pract. 2021;75:e14135.
14. Saud A, Naveen R, Aggarwal R, Gupta L. COVID-19 and myositis: what we know so far. Curr Rheumatol Rep. 2021;23:63.
15. Hassan M, Ullah Khan N, Iqbal Chaudhary M, Jan Z, Majid Rajput H, Susan Dewey R, Badshah M. Neurological complications of SARS CoV 2: a single-center case series. Brain Hemorrhages. 2021;2(4):161–4. https://doi.org/10.1016/j.hest.2021.09.004.

16. Deeb A, Kumar PC, Sakrani N, Trehan RK, Papinenei VR. Neurological presentations of COVID-19: characteristic features in a case series of hospitalized patients from Abu Dhabi, UAE. BioMed Res Int. 2021;2021:5822259.
17. Gokhale Y, Patankar A, Holla U, Shilke M, Kalekar L, Karnik ND, Bidichandani K, Baveja S, Joshi A. Dermatomyositis during COVID-19 pandemic (a case series): is there a cause effect relationship? J Assoc Physicians India. 2020;68:20–4.
18. Rebendenne A, Valadão ALC, Tauziet M, et al. SARS-CoV-2 triggers an MDA-5-dependent interferon response which is unable to control replication in lung epithelial cells. J Virol. 2021;95(8):e02415–20.
19. Aschman T, Schneider J, Greuel S, et al. Association between SARS-CoV-2 infection and immune-mediated myopathy in patients who have died. JAMA Neurol. 2021;78:948–60.
20. Dalakas MC. Unconvincing evidence of SARS-CoV-2-associated myositis in autopsied muscles. JAMA Neurol. 2021;79(1):92–3. https://doi.org/10.1001/jamaneurol.2021.4336.
21. Mehan WA, Yoon BC, Lang M, Li MD, Rincon S, Buch K. Paraspinal myositis in patients with COVID-19 infection. AJNR Am J Neuroradiol. 2020;41:1949–52.
22. Armstrong BK, Murchison AP, Bilyk JR. Suspected orbital myositis associated with COVID-19. Orbit. 2021;40(6):532–5. https://doi.org/10.1080/01676830.2021.1962366.
23. Almadani M, Shiferson A, Swearingen B, Shih M, Jacob T, Rhee R. Compartment syndrome secondary to viral myositis as initial presentation in COVID-19 patient. J Vasc Surg Cases Innov Tech. 2020;6:524–7.
24. Kumar NB. Does COVID-19-related cachexia mimic cancer-related cachexia? Examining mechanisms, clinical biomarkers, and potential targets for clinical management. J Cachexia Sarcopenia Muscle. 2021;12:519–22.
25. Bahouth S, Chuang K, Olson L, Rosenthal D. COVID-19 related muscle denervation atrophy. Skelet Radiol. 2021;50:1717–21.
26. Becker RC. COVID-19-associated vasculitis and vasculopathy. J Thromb Thrombolysis. 2020;50:499–511.
27. Colmenero I, Santonja C, Alonso-Riaño M, Noguera-Morel L, Hernández-Martín A, Andina D, Wiesner T, Rodríguez-Peralto JL, Requena L, Torrelo A. SARS-CoV-2 endothelial infection causes COVID-19 chilblains: histopathological, immunohistochemical and ultrastructural study of seven paediatric cases. Br J Dermatol. 2020;183:729–37.
28. Kumar G, Pillai S, Norwick P, Bukulmez H. Leucocytoclastic vasculitis secondary to COVID-19 infection in a young child. BMJ Case Rep. 2021;14:e242192.
29. Kashi M, Jacquin A, Dakhil B, Zaimi R, Mahé E, Tella E, Bagan P. Severe arterial thrombosis associated with Covid-19 infection. Thromb Res. 2020;192:75–7.
30. Quintana-Castanedo L, Feito-Rodríguez M, Fernández-Alcalde C, Granados-Fernández M, Montero-Vega D, Mayor-Ibarguren A, de Lucas-Laguna R. Concurrent chilblains and retinal vasculitis in a child with COVID-19. J Eur Acad Dermatol Venereol. 2020;34:e764–6.
31. Vulliamy P, Jacob S, Davenport RA. Acute aorto-iliac and mesenteric arterial thromboses as presenting features of COVID-19. Br J Haematol. 2020;189:1053–4.
32. Menter T, Haslbauer JD, Nienhold R, et al. Postmortem examination of COVID-19 patients reveals diffuse alveolar damage with severe capillary congestion and variegated findings in lungs and other organs suggesting vascular dysfunction. Histopathology. 2020;77:198–209.
33. Pinto AA, Carroll LS, Nar V, Varatharaj A, Galea I. CNS inflammatory vasculopathy with antimyelin oligodendrocyte glycoprotein antibodies in COVID-19. Neurol Neuroimmunol Neuroinflamm. 2020;7:e813.
34. Camprodon Gómez M, González-Cruz C, Ferrer B, Barberá MJ. Leucocytoclastic vasculitis in a patient with COVID-19 with positive SARS-CoV-2 PCR in skin biopsy. BMJ Case Rep. 2020;13:e238039.
35. Kant S, Raman G, Damera P, Antiochos B, Seo P, Geetha D. Characteristics and outcomes of COVID-19 in patients with antineutrophil cytoplasmic antibody-associated vasculitis. Kidney Int Rep. 2021;6:806–9.

36. Uppal NN, Kello N, Shah HH, Khanin Y, De Oleo IR, Epstein E, Sharma P, Larsen CP, Bijol V, Jhaveri KD. De novo ANCA-associated vasculitis with glomerulonephritis in COVID-19. Kidney Int Rep. 2020;5:2079–83.
37. Lecler A, Villeneuve D, Vignal C, Sené T. Increased rather than decreased incidence of giant-cell arteritis during the COVID-19 pandemic. Ann Rheum Dis. 2020;80(6):e89.
38. Luther R, Skeoch S, Pauling JD, Curd C, Woodgate F, Tansley S. Increased number of cases of giant cell arteritis and higher rates of ophthalmic involvement during the era of COVID-19. Rheumatol Adv Pract. 2020;4:rkaa067.
39. Parreau S, Liozon E, Ly K-H, Fauchais A-L, Hantz S. High incidence of giant cell arteritis during the COVID-19 pandemic: no causal relationship but possible involvement of stress. Clin Exp Rheumatol. 2021;39(Suppl 129):199–200.
40. Mehta P, Sattui SE, van der Geest KSM, Brouwer E, Conway R, Putman MS, Robinson PC, Mackie SL. Giant cell arteritis and COVID-19: similarities and discriminators. A systematic literature review. J Rheumatol. 2021;48:1053–9.
41. Harzallah I, Debliquis A, Drénou B. Lupus anticoagulant is frequent in patients with Covid-19. J Thromb Haemost. 2020;18:2064–5.
42. Fan BE, Ng J, Chan SSW, et al. COVID-19 associated coagulopathy in critically ill patients: a hypercoagulable state demonstrated by parameters of haemostasis and clot waveform analysis. J Thromb Thrombolysis. 2021;51:663–74.
43. Connell NT, Battinelli EM, Connors JM. Coagulopathy of COVID-19 and antiphospholipid antibodies. J Thromb Haemost. 2020; https://doi.org/10.1111/jth.14893.
44. Favaloro EJ, Henry BM, Lippi G. COVID-19 and Antiphospholipid antibodies: time for a reality check? Semin Thromb Hemost. 2021;48(1):72–92. https://doi.org/10.1055/s-0041-1728832.
45. Schofield JR. Persistent antiphospholipid antibodies, mast cell activation syndrome, postural orthostatic tachycardia syndrome and post-COVID syndrome. 1 year on. Eur J Case Rep Intern Med. 2021;8:002378.
46. Johansson M, Ståhlberg M, Runold M, Nygren-Bonnier M, Nilsson J, Olshansky B, Bruchfeld J, Fedorowski A. Long-haul post-COVID-19 symptoms presenting as a variant of postural orthostatic tachycardia syndrome: the Swedish experience. JACC Case Rep. 2021;3:573–80.
47. Bertin D, Kaphan E, Weber S, Babacci B, Arcani R, Faucher B, Ménard A, Brodovitch A, Mege JL, Bardin N. Persistent IgG anticardiolipin autoantibodies are associated with post-COVID syndrome. Int J Infect Dis. 2021;113:23–5.
48. Wong SW, Fan BE, Huang W, Chia YW. ST-segment elevation myocardial infarction in post-COVID-19 patients: a case series. Ann Acad Med Singap. 2021;50:425–30.
49. Ramos-Casals M, Brito-Zerón P, Mariette X. Systemic and organ-specific immune-related manifestations of COVID-19. Nat Rev Rheumatol. 2021;17:315–32.
50. Zacharias H, Dubey S, Koduri G, D'Cruz D. Rheumatological complications of Covid 19. Autoimmun Rev. 2021;20:102883.
51. Slimani Y, Abbassi R, El Fatoiki F-Z, Barrou L, Chiheb S. Systemic lupus erythematosus and varicella-like rash following COVID-19 in a previously healthy patient. J Med Virol. 2021;93:1184–7.
52. Zamani B, Moeini Taba S-M, Shayestehpour M. Systemic lupus erythematosus manifestation following COVID-19: a case report. J Med Case Rep. 2021;15:29.
53. Shayestehpour M, Zamani B. The first case of systemic lupus erythematosus (SLE) triggered by COVID-19 infection. Eur Rev Med Pharmacol Sci. 2020;24:11474.
54. Bonometti R, Sacchi MC, Stobbione P, et al. The first case of systemic lupus erythematosus (SLE) triggered by COVID-19 infection. Eur Rev Med Pharmacol Sci. 2020;24:9695–7.
55. Li Z-X, Zeng S, Wu H-X, Zhou Y. The risk of systemic lupus erythematosus associated with Epstein-Barr virus infection: a systematic review and meta-analysis. Clin Exp Med. 2019;19:23–36.
56. Gianfrancesco M, Hyrich KL, Al-Adely S, et al. Characteristics associated with hospitalisation for COVID 19 in people with rheumatic disease: data from the COVID-19 Global Rheumatology Alliance physician-reported registry. Ann Rheum Dis. 2020;79:859–66.

57. Williamson EJ, Walker AJ, Bhaskaran K, et al. Factors associated with COVID-19-related death using OpenSAFELY. Nature. 2020;584:430–6.
58. Akiyama S, Hamdeh S, Micic D, Sakuraba A. Prevalence and clinical outcomes of COVID-19 in patients with autoimmune diseases: a systematic review and meta-analysis. Ann Rheum Dis. 2020;80(3):384–91.

12 Dermatological Sequelae of COVID-19 Infection

Pankhuri Dudani, Vishal Gupta, and Kaushal K. Verma

12.1 Introduction

Cutaneous involvement in patients with COVID-19 infection has been reported to range from 0.2 to 45% in different hospital-based studies from India and abroad. A population-based patient-reported survey of 336,847 patients from the UK found 21% of COVID-19-positive patients reporting skin features as the *only* symptom of COVID-19 infection, while the skin manifestations preceded other symptoms in 17% of patients [1]. Patient-reported studies from Thailand [2], France [3], and Turkey [4] have shown a frequency of 15% ($n = 183$), 1% ($n = 756$), and 18.3% ($n = 382$) of cutaneous lesions; lower frequencies, 1.5% ($n = 130$) in Italy [5], 4.3% ($n = 69$) in Japan [6], and 7.25% ($n = 138$) in India [7], were reported in studies with in-person examination by dermatologists. More recently, a Spanish study in hospitalized patients reported an incidence of 3.5% ($n = 144$) [8], while 2 cross-sectional observational studies from tertiary-care centers in Northern India including 1659 asymptomatic/mildly symptomatic and 270 moderate/severe COVID-19 disease reported a much lower incidence of 0.6% and 2.59%, respectively [9, 10]. Two systematic reviews on cutaneous manifestations of COVID-19 have reported an incidence of 5.69 and 5.95%, respectively [11, 12]. In addition, a case-control study from Austria (cases, n = 103; controls, n = 41) did not report a statistically significant difference between confirmed cases of COVID 19 and controls who had other acute infectious diseases [13]. They suggested that the cutaneous involvement in COVID-19 is not specific and does not have diagnostic value. The true incidence may be closer to that reported in the later studies; reasons for a lower incidence in these studies include in-person evaluation by a dermatologist, a better understanding of the cutaneous involvement and attribution to COVID-19 by the

P. Dudani · V. Gupta · K. K. Verma (✉)
Department of Dermatology and Venereology, AIIMS, New Delhi, India

A. Mohan, S. Mittal (eds.), *Post COVID-19 Complications and Management*, https://doi.org/10.1007/978-981-19-4407-9_12

investigators, and more robust investigations to rule out other causes. A systematic review for prognostic value of the cutaneous manifestations reported that urticaria-like lesions had the least mortality (2.2%) while livedo/purpuric lesions were associated with the highest mortality rate (18.2%) [11].

12.2 Dermatological Manifestations of COVID-19 Infection

Common dermatological manifestations associated with COVID-19 infection are summarized in Table 12.1. The involvement of any organ by COVID-19 is determined by the expression of viral receptors, which include ACE-2 (angiotensin-converting enzyme 2) and TMPRSS2 (transmembrane protease serine 2) [15]. The former is highly expressed in alveolar cells of the lungs, explaining the virtually universal involvement of lungs.

The virus cannot penetrate and infect the skin primarily (though the keratinocytes express both ACE-2 and TMPRSS2 receptors); all skin manifestations are indirect in nature as a result of blood-borne dissemination (ACE-2 is expressed in capillary endothelial cells) [15]. The pathogenesis of the skin manifestations is unclear; a simplified classification divides them into "inflammatory" lesions which form due to aberrant immune responses to viral components (maculopapular lesions, urticaria, vesicular lesions) and "vascular" secondary to vasculopathy and thrombotic phenomena (erythema pernio-like, livedo, purpuric lesions) [16]. The viral spike protein has been demonstrated in skin lesions in multiple studies, even in the

Table 12.1 Summary of common dermatological manifestations with temporal correlation, frequency of occurrence, and association with severity of systemic COVID-19 disease [11, 12]

Cutaneous manifestation	Onset	Persistence up to	Frequency/ incidence (%)	Severity of COVID-19 infection
Maculopapular	Before other symptoms, as late as 4 weeks after resolution of symptoms [14]	7–14 days	36–48	Mild
Urticarial	Before, up to 2 weeks after other symptoms	4–28 days	9–15	Mild
Pseudochilblains / erythema pernio-like	2 weeks after other symptoms	Up to 150 days (Average, 15 days)	18–51	Mild or asymptomatic
Vesicular/ vesiculobullous	Before, or up to 1 week after other symptoms	90 days	9–15	Mild to moderate
Livedo/purpura/ necrosis	2–4 weeks after other symptoms	Up to 150 days	4–9	Severe
Acute telogen effluvium	6 weeks after diagnosis	36 weeks	30–50	In all grades of severity

absence of PCR positivity in nasal swab samples [17]. Virus-induced endothelial damage has been observed in some skin biopsies from pernio-like lesions, which supports the causal association of these lesions with COVID-19 [18]. However, viral proteins are not always detectable in skin tissue samples, and some studies suggest that reactivation of latent HHV-6 infection may be responsible for some observations such as maculopapular rash, pityriasis rosea lesions, and DRESS (drug reaction with eosinophilia and systemic symptoms)-like lesions.

While current data allows a rough timeline to be constructed with most skin changes developing within 4 weeks from onset of other COVID-19 symptoms, delayed manifestations of skin lesions have also been observed and reported. This precludes temporal correlation from being used as a strict criterion for COVID-19-related skin changes, and does not allow a strict differentiation between manifestations of COVID-19 infection and post-COVID-19 changes.

12.2.1 Skin Changes

Maculopapular rash is the most frequent cutaneous manifestation of COVID-19 according to most systematic reviews (36–48%) and consists of erythematous macules and papules in a generalized distribution, which may initially be discrete and later coalesce (Fig. 12.1) [11, 12]. Other morphologies included within this term are pityriasis rosea-like and erythema multiforme-like changes [19]. The skin lesions usually start within 2-10 days of other symptoms of COVID-19 infection, some reports have noted a delayed onset of 4 weeks also. These lesions are associated with mild COVID-19 disease in 48% of cases which usually does not require any intervention, and resolve in 7–10 days [11].

Pernio-like lesions/pseudochilblains, the next most common manifestation (18–51%), are described as persistent redness of the periungual region, also called "COVID toes." Rarely, there may be associated pustulation and crusting. These have been noted more frequently in children, young adults, and elderly individuals (Fig. 12.2) and may be the sole manifestation of COVID-19 infection. They are mostly associated with mild disease (82%). They may be the only presenting feature in 10–15% of cases and may precede other symptoms in another 10% of cases; in most cases they start within 2 weeks of other symptoms, last up to 2 weeks, and require no active intervention. Rarely, they may last longer (reported up to 150 days) and may be associated with dysesthesia.

Urticarial lesions, presenting as itchy red wheals (Fig. 12.3), are usually generalized in distribution and rarely associated with angioedema. They are rarer, seen in 9–15% of COVID-19 patients with cutaneous lesions, mostly associated with mild disease (51–53%). These may precede other COVID-19 symptoms by 1–2 days (5–6%) and, thus, might be the presenting feature of COVID-19 [11, 12]. The urticarial condition lasts for 7–10 days while being treated with antihistamines with/without low-dose systemic corticosteroids. Rarely, they may persist for a month.

Vesiculobullous lesions consist of fluid-filled lesions in a localized or generalized distribution, often sparing the mucosa. When generalized, they appear varicella-like

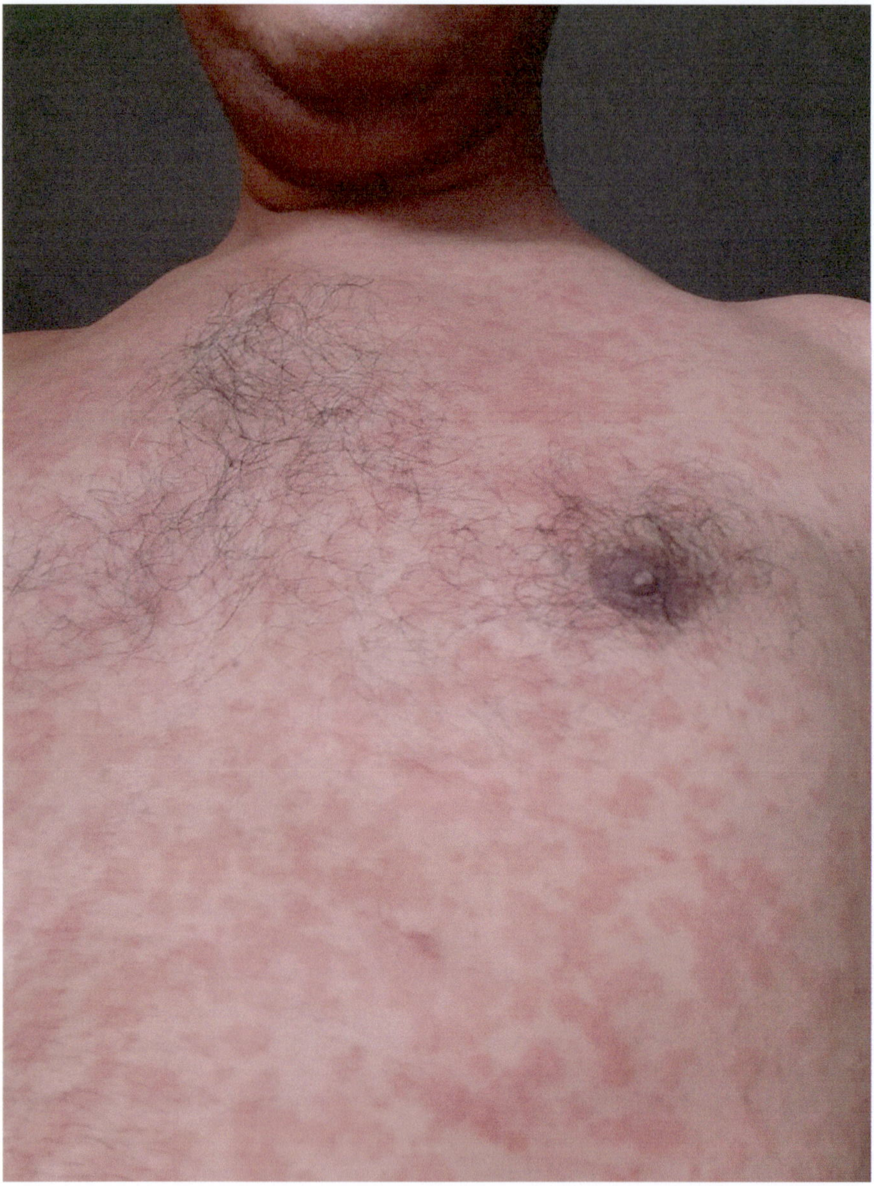

Fig. 12.1 Maculopapular rash in an adult male patient with COVID-19 infection

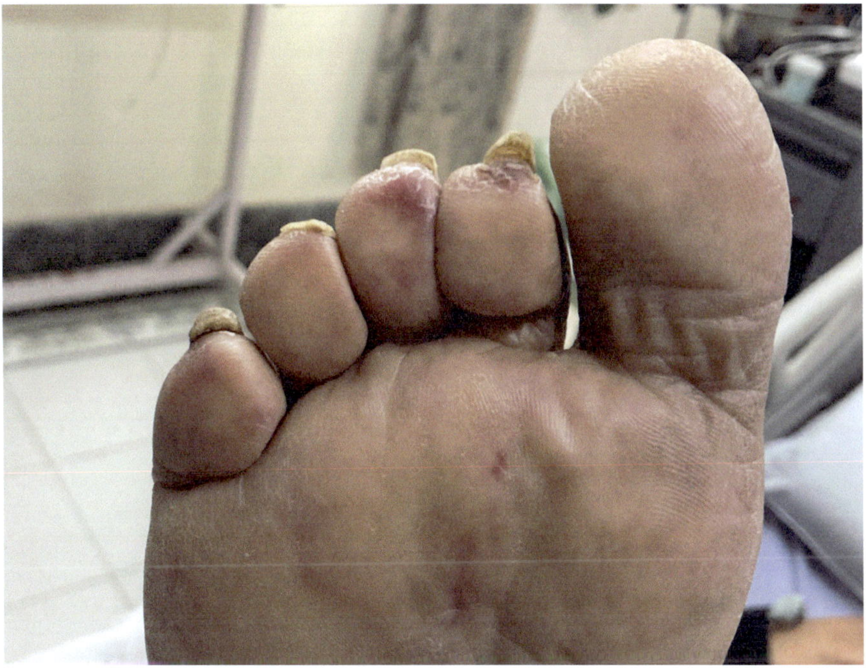

Fig. 12.2 Pseudochilblains in an elderly patient, 6 weeks after recovery from COVID-19 infection

and may involve the palms and soles. They are seen in 9–15% of cases, about half of them with mild COVID-19 disease. These lesions usually start within 3 days and last up to 7–10 days. Herpetic infections may have to be ruled out in some cases depending on morphology and distribution of lesions, e.g., in herpes zoster, they are in a dermatomal distribution, while in herpes simplex they are closely grouped and may coalesce.

Livedo or retiform purpura manifests as localized or diffuse red-purple non-blanchable discoloration of the skin, especially over acral sites. This may form a network and later develop ulceration. They are observed in 4–9% of patients with skin manifestations of COVID-19, most often in association with severe COVID-19 features. These are important to be noted as they are associated with other thrombotic events and a higher mortality rate (15–18%) [11, 19]. This might be due to the same mechanism of formation of these lesions and end-organ damage to the other systems, i.e., microangiopathy secondary to an altered thrombotic pathway.

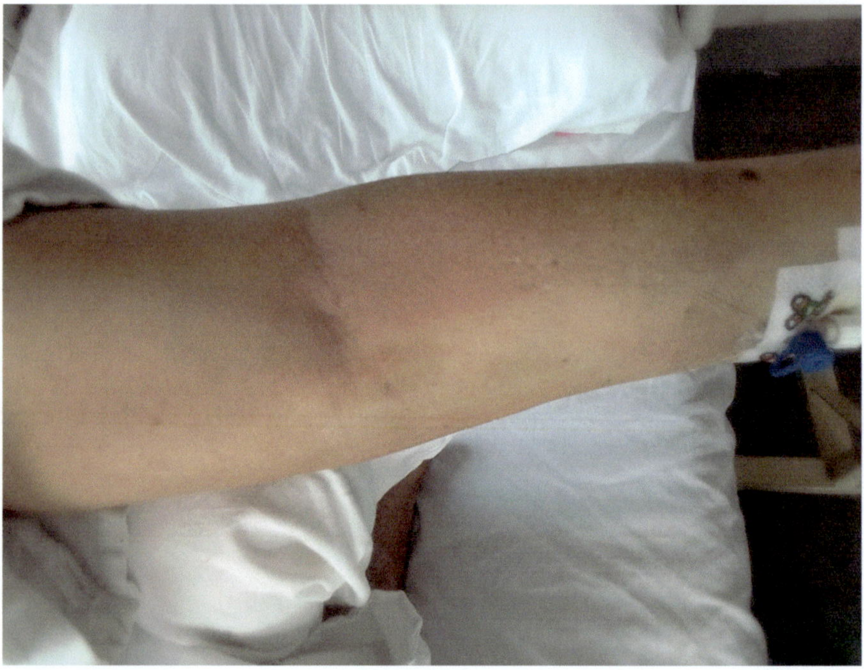

Fig. 12.3 Transient urticarial lesion over the cubital fossa in a 19-year-old male patient (*Image courtesy of Dr Rashi Pangti, Department of Dermatology and Venereology, AIIMS, New Delhi*)

Multisystem inflammatory syndrome in adults (>*21 years*) *and children* (<*21 years*), also known as Kawasaki-like disease, is a rare but serious post-COVID-19 manifestation. The patients present with persistent fever, generalized skin lesions, mucositis (including conjunctivitis), acral edema, erythema and desquamation, gastrointestinal symptoms (abdominal pain, vomiting, diarrhea), neurocognitive symptoms (headache, confusion, lethargy), and respiratory symptoms [20]. The morphology of skin lesions is variable, including maculopapular, urticarial (Fig. 12.4), purpuric (Fig. 12.5), and even erythroderma. These symptoms may start up to few weeks to months following COVID-19; the latter may have been asymptomatic or mild disease. Compared to Kawasaki disease, this syndrome is seen in older patients, has cutaneous manifestations more often (30 vs. 70%), and has a more rapid and severe deterioration of systemic status [21].

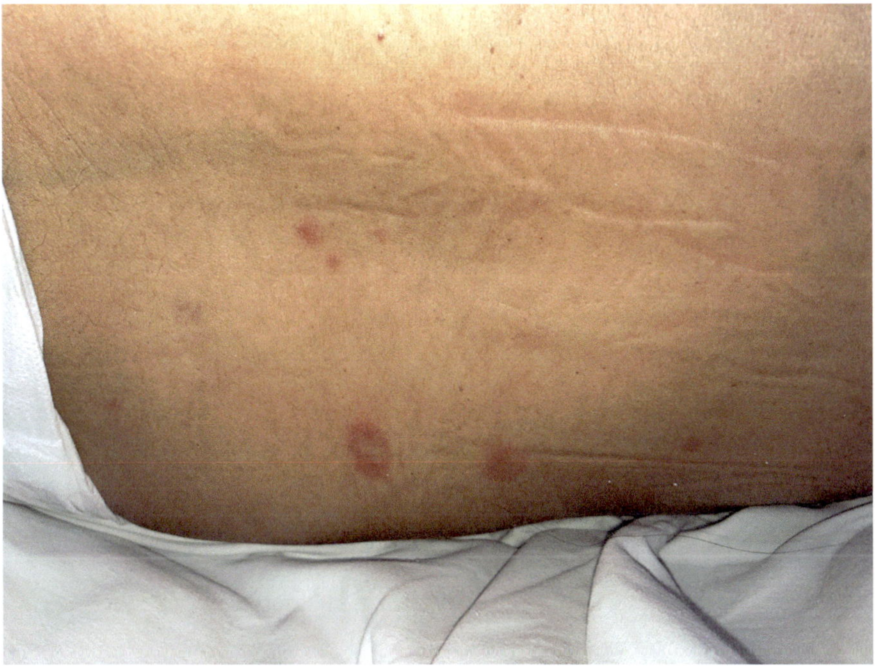

Fig. 12.4 Urticarial vasculitis-like lesions on the trunk of an adult patient with post-COVID-19 multisystem inflammatory syndrome

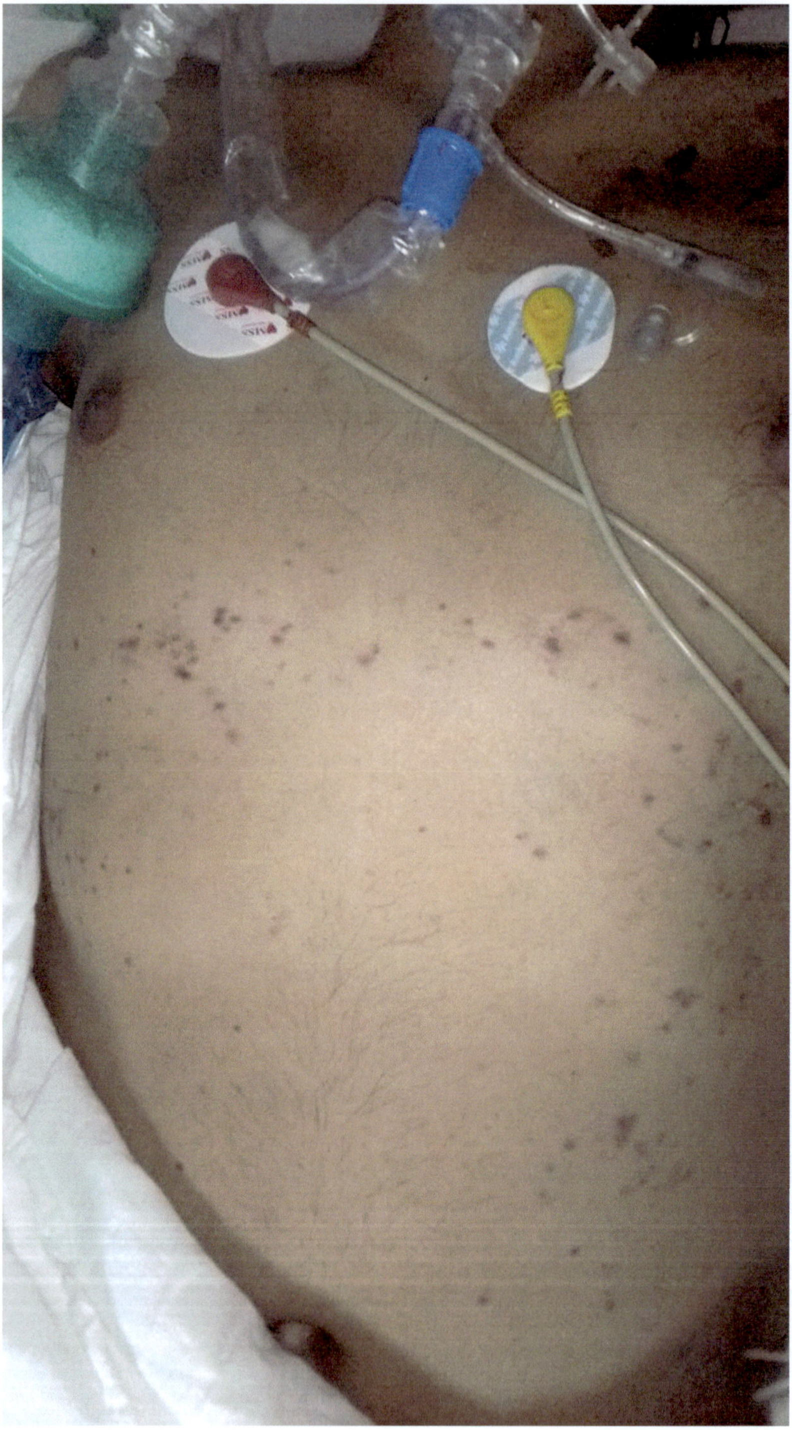

Fig. 12.5 Dusky erythematous (purpuric) macules and papules on the trunk of a critically ill patient with severe COVID-19 infection

12.2.2 Trigger or Exacerbation of Skin Diseases

Flaring up of previously controlled or subsided autoimmune diseases has been noted in patients with lichen planus (Fig. 12.6), psoriasis (Fig. 12.7), atopic dermatitis, seborrheic dermatitis, and acne [19].

Herpes zoster reactivation may occur up to 6 weeks post-COVID-19 infection (Fig. 12.8); however, it may even precede the symptoms by 2–3 days. The treatment remains the same with systemic antivirals (acyclovir/valacyclovir) for 7–10 days.

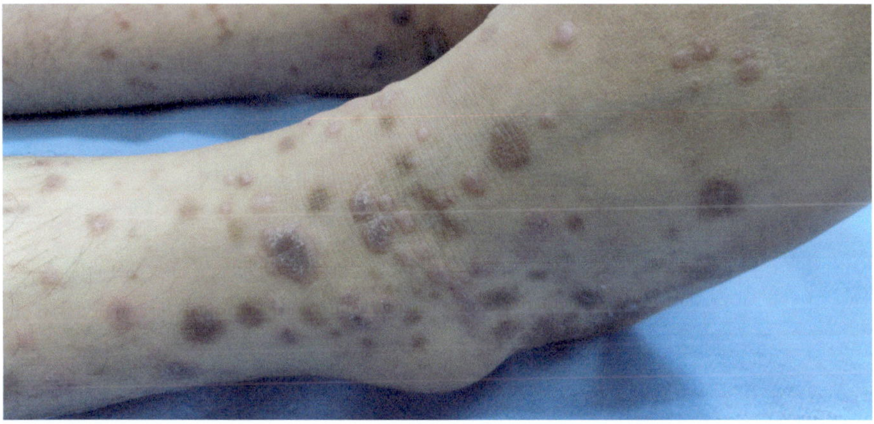

Fig. 12.6 Eruptive lichen planus lesions over the dorsa of ankles in a known case of lichen planus, 3 weeks post-COVID-19 infection (*Image courtesy of Dr Vishal Gaurav*). Older lesions have subsided with post-inflammatory hyperpigmentation

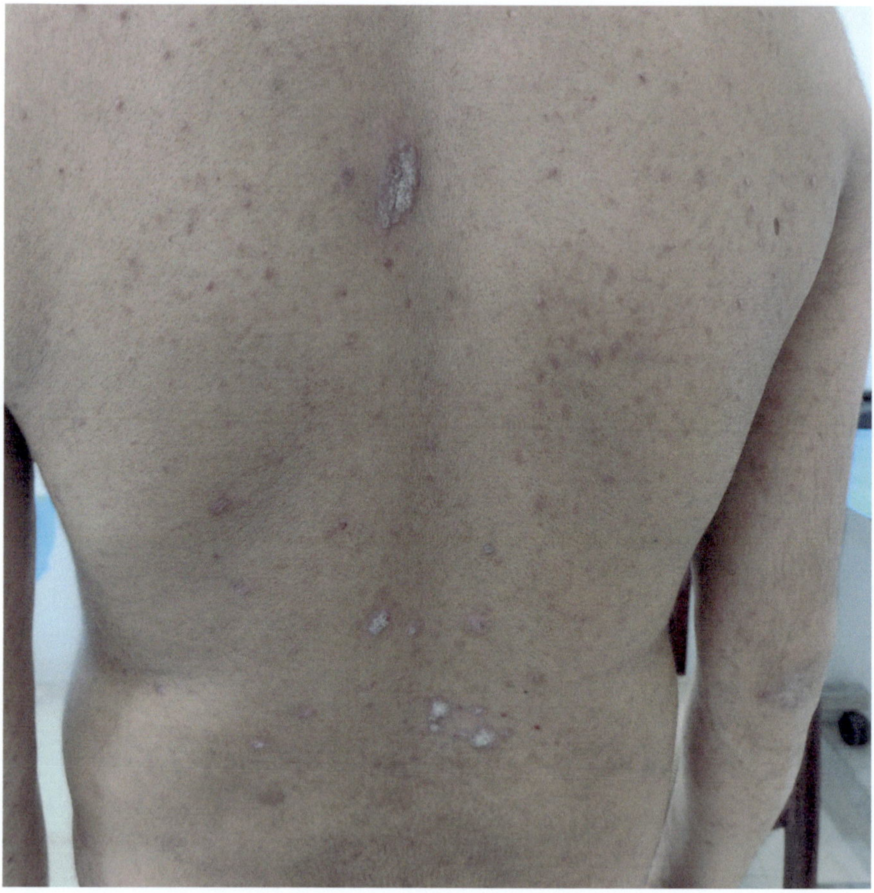

Fig. 12.7 Multiple psoriasis lesions appearing over the trunk in a patient with previously controlled disease; 2 weeks post-COVID-19 infection (*Image courtesy of Dr Vishal Gaurav, Department of Dermatology and Venereology, AIIMS, New Delhi*)

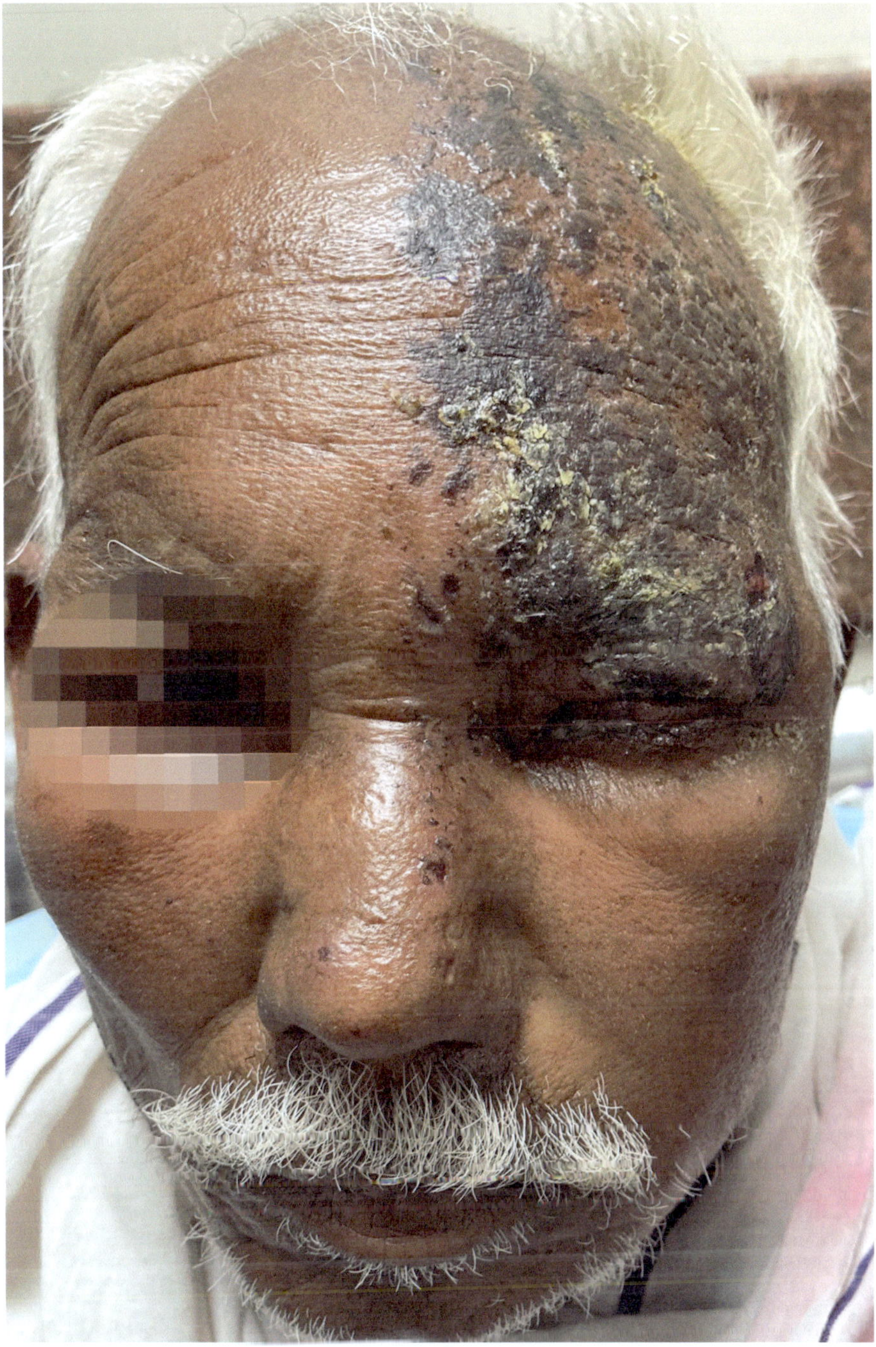

Fig. 12.8 Herpes zoster ophthalmicus in a 60 year-old male patient, 10 days after diagnosis of COVID-19

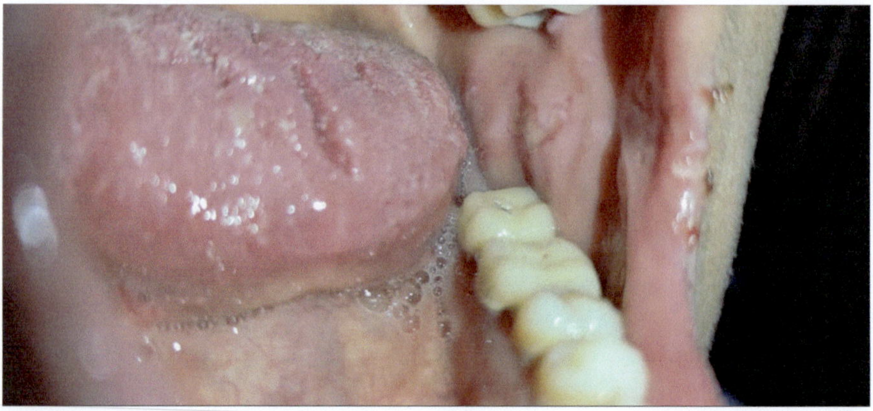

Fig. 12.9 Multiple fissures over the dorsum of the tongue, left angle of the mouth, an aphthous ulcer over left buccal mucosa in a 59-year-old female patient, 2 weeks after diagnosis of COVID-19

12.2.3 Mucosal Manifestations

Mucosal changes are rarely observable in COVID-19 patients; while there are no studies yet on the prevalence of mucosal manifestations in COVID-19 patients, an international registry of skin and mucosal manifestations in 716 patients from 31 countries reported mucosal lesions to be seen in about 5% of those reporting skin/mucosal manifestations [22]. Hence, mucosal sites must always be examined in patients of COVID-19. Patients may demonstrate hyperemia of the oral mucosa, single-to-few aphthous ulcers, depapillation of the tongue, fissures over the angles of the mouth, and frank necrosis of buccal mucosa [23] (Fig. 12.9). In addition, oral lichen planus may be triggered de novo by COVID-19 infection; however, the correlation is not strong, and the data is limited to case reports.

12.2.4 Hair

Hair loss and scalp symptoms, both localized and generalized, have been observed in relation to COVID-19 infection. A majority are reported after weeks of COVID-19 infection, although an early onset has been occasionally observed.

Acute telogen effluvium is a self-limited diffuse loss of hair which occurs 2–3 months after a stressful triggering event such as major surgery, postpartum, and prolonged or high-grade fever such as seen in malaria typhoid and lupus. The precipitating event causes premature termination of anagen phase and conversion to catagen and subsequently telogen phases. COVID-19 infection causes a systemic inflammatory response and this proinflammatory state may cause telogen effluvium [24–27]. Tumor necrosis factor-α, IFN types 1 and 2, IL-6, MMP-1 and MMP-3, and IL-1β have been hypothesized to play a role, in addition to microthrombi formation and direct damage to the hair follicle by the virus after entry into the basal keratinocytes (via the ACE-2 and TMPRSS2 receptors) [28]. The patients present with sudden increase in hair loss, including hair coming out in clumps and thinning seen over the frontal hairline about 6–7 weeks after RT-PCR positivity or other symptoms of COVID-19. In a prospective study of 204 SARS-CoV-2-positive patients in Turkey including equal numbers of admitted patients and outpatients with COVID-19-related symptoms, acute telogen effluvium was noted in about one-fourth of COVID-19 patients, with majority being females (65–70%) [29]. The incidence in mild versus hospitalized groups was comparable, with 24% of patients with mild disease and 31% of patients in hospitalized group. The onset was noted at 6–7 weeks after RT-PCR positivity (earliest at 4 weeks) and lasted for a median of 47.5 days after onset (range, 12–100 days). COVID-19 infection-associated telogen effluvium was noted to be more intense, earlier in onset, and earlier to resolve than acute telogen effluvium due to other causes, possibly due to direct follicular damage by the virus [29]. Management is expectant, as it is a self-resolving condition. Agents such as topical minoxidil (5%) and oral multivitamins may be used; however, *reassurance* is the key intervention. Some case reports of acute anagen effluvium and alopecia areata also exist, but larger studies are required to confirm a causal association.

Trichodynia encompasses multiple symptoms like itching, burning, pain, or paresthesia in the scalp, with or without accompanying telogen effluvium. It can start early and is seen in more than half the patients with COVID-19 infection presenting to dermatologists and may be underreported due to its variable and nonserious nature. It correlates with increased neuropeptide substance P expression. Helpful interventions include adequate sleep, washing scalp with warm water, and topical corticosteroids; however, it may last for months and patients may require repeated sessions of counselling [24].

12.2.5 Nail

Nail plate changes can be seen in about 1% of patients with COVID-19 infection, although these may be underreported as prevalence studies are lacking. They usually follow the disease or insult by a few weeks as it takes time for the altered nail plate to emerge from under the proximal nail fold; however, vascular changes can appear early, during COVID-19 infection, similar to systemic vascular manifestations [30–32]. The red half-moon nail sign, possibly pathognomonic for COVID-19 infection, consists of distally convex red bands, placed just distal to the lunula, over multiple fingernails. This manifestation might be due to microvascular injury to the distal subungual capillary network as a part of systemic inflammatory response, similar to that seen in Kawasaki disease. It is seen as early as 2 days prior to the onset of other symptoms, even though it may start later within 2 weeks. These changes may persist for 1–6 weeks after onset [33].

Mees' lines are transverse leukonychia (white lines) in all nail plates, noted 3–6 weeks (maximum 16 weeks) after onset of other symptoms of COVID-19. It is due to altered keratinization of the nail plate due to temporary dysfunction of the nail matrix as a consequence of systemic illness. These are non-blanchable and grow out with time, in about 4–6 weeks.

Beau's lines are transverse *grooves* in the nail plate due to temporary suspension of keratinization following acute stress to the nail matrix, visible about 2–3 weeks after the acute event once nail plate growth is resumed. If the nail plate keratinization is arrested completely, it leads to *onychomadesis*, i.e., a nail plate which is completely separated from the nail matrix while remaining attached to the nail bed. Both these changes are also self-limited as the nail grows out normally after the systemic insult is over [31, 32].

Periungual desquamation is seen at the proximal and lateral nail folds and has been seen in children with severe Kawasaki-like multisystem inflammatory syndrome (MIS-C) and adults with severe COVID-19 infection at the time of recovery [32].

12.3 Skin Involvement due to Agents Used in Treatment of COVID-19 Infection

The treatment of COVID-19 infection depends on severity of the disease and includes a wide gamut of medications with variable efficacy which lead to either direct changes on the skin or skin changes secondary to altered physiology induced by the medications [34]. Discontinuation of the drug is warranted only in the case of severe cutaneous adverse drug reactions, for example, acute generalized exanthematous pustulosis (AGEP), drug reaction with eosinophilia and systemic symptoms (DRESS), and Stevens-Johnson syndrome/toxic epidermal necrolysis. Hydroxychloroquine use can lead to pigmentary effects such as longitudinal pigmented bands in multiple nails, generalized hyperpigmentation, and graying of hair in up to a third of the patients; other adverse effects include hypersensitivity reactions such as maculopapular rash, acute generalized exanthematous pustulosis, drug reaction with eosinophilia and systemic symptoms, erythema multiforme, and Stevens-Johnson syndrome. Systemic corticosteroids are known to lead to cutaneous adverse effects in a majority (10–70%) of patients, such as striae, telangiectasias, hypertrichosis, and acneiform eruption. Remdesivir, the antiviral agent, can cause a generalized self-limited maculopapular rash in up to 7% of recipients, as well as another cutaneous adverse eruption called symmetrical drug-related intertriginous and flexural exanthema, which involves confluent erythematous maculopapular lesions over the flexures and buttocks. Darunavir, another antiviral agent, has been associated with maculopapular, vesicular, and purpuric lesions, as well as rare reports of SJS, the former in up to 10% of patients [34]. Favipiravir has been associated with observation of a yellow-white or green fluorescence of nails and hair seen on Wood's lamp examination, possibly due to metabolites of the excipient ferric oxide in the tablets. Ribavirin has been associated with induced alopecia and photoallergic reaction in up to a fifth of patients, while interferons can cause induced urticaria and even generalized eczematous changes. Tocilizumab can cause multiple cutaneous adverse events such as maculopapular rash (up to 10% of patients), urticaria, AGEP, DRESS, and SJS. Immunoglobulin infusion is associated with urticaria during infusion, as well as delayed manifestation of maculopapular rash and erythema multiforme. Low-molecular-weight heparin can rarely (<1% of recipients) cause heparin-induced skin necrosis. Lastly, noninvasive ventilation may lead to pressure ulcers and even prolonged xerostomia [35].

12.4 Skin Changes due to Use of Personal Protective Equipment

Use of personal protective equipment leads to buildup of secretions (sweat) along with prolonged friction. The damage to skin barrier is multiplied due to use of sanitizers and other disinfecting agents. This also increases the chances of developing irritant and allergic contact dermatitis to the constituents of the protective equipment (Fig. 12.10a, b). In self-reported questionnaire-based studies, 70–88% of frontline healthcare workers reported adverse skin reactions, the most common being nasal-bridge inflammation and scarring, indentation and inflammation behind the ears, and excessive sweating within double-latex gloves [36]. Use of PPE longer than 6 h/day and working more than 3 days a week were associated with adverse skin changes [36, 37].

An ideal mask should have no metallic part at the bridge of the nose and have adjustable draw strings to allow one size to fit all, with the adjustable bead being *flat*. After wearing, the mask should allow air movement while speaking. An ill-fitting mask can induce acne, or “maskne,” noted over the area covered by the mask, newly referred to as the “O” zone of the face (Fig. 12.11) [38]. The friction and changed skin microenvironment, i.e., increased heat and humidity leading to altered microbiome, are hypothesized to play a role. Management includes antibiotic washes and hydrogel formulations of retinoids. Spot application of conventional

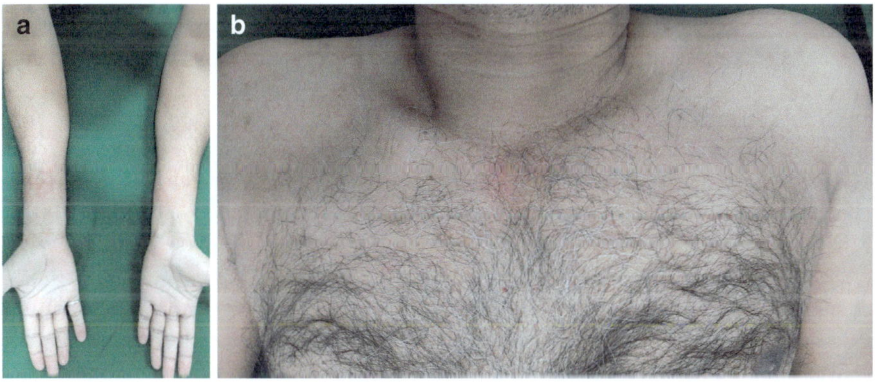

Fig. 12.10 (**a**, **b**) Allergic contact dermatitis to textile/washing agent in a healthcare worker. Erythematous, edematous papules at the site of maximum friction with scrubs (neckline, elastic sleeve cuff) (*Images courtesy of Dr Ananya Sharma, Department of Dermatology and Venereology, AIIMS, New Delhi*)

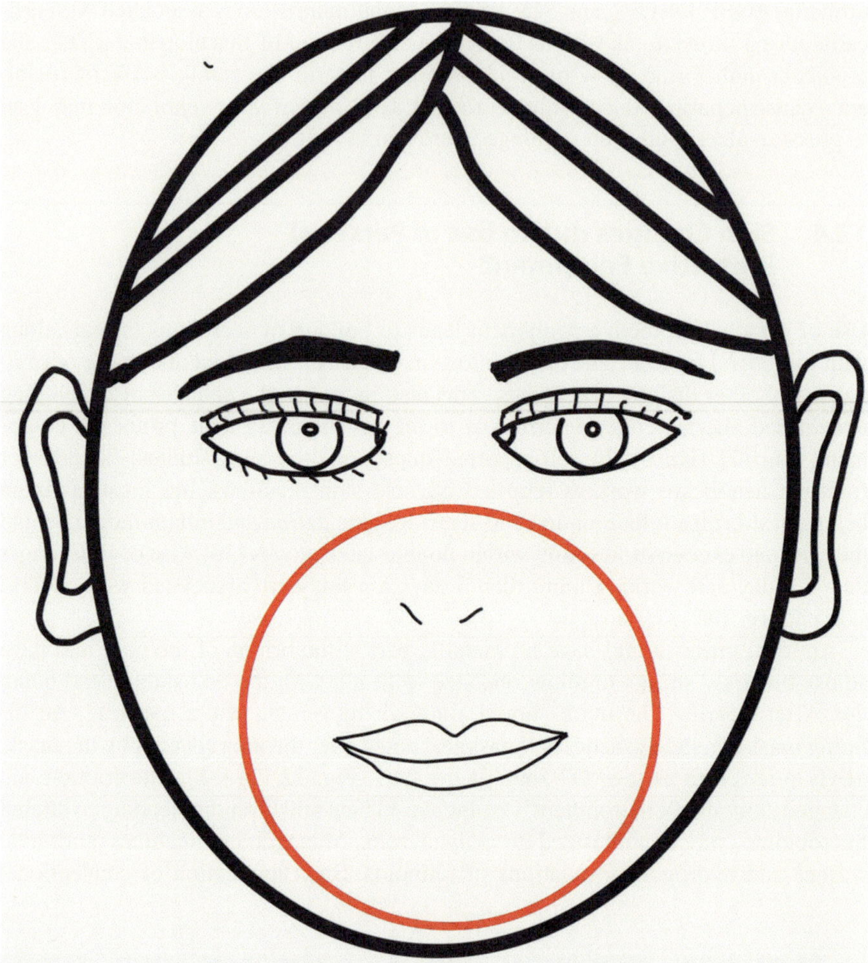

Fig. 12.11 Schematic diagram showing the newly described "O" zone of the face, along the margins and within which acneiform eruptions induced by a mask are likely to form

acne agents is *not* recommended as it may cause irritation if occluded by the mask after application [39]. Allergic contact dermatitis may occur due to sensitization to zinc released from metallic part over the nose. Latex or the accelerants used in elastic ear loops may also lead to contact dermatitis of eczematous or noneczematous type over the retroauricular regions and nape of the neck (Fig. 12.12a, b); similar changes may occur over the hands due to use of latex gloves. Pressure-induced abrasion and ulceration over the bridge of the nose and cheeks due to continued localized trauma by the mask are seen; similar changes may be seen over the forehead due to use of the face shield.

Hand-washing and alcohol-based sanitization measures lead to continued disruption of the natural lipid skin barrier and result in "COVID hand dermatitis." The

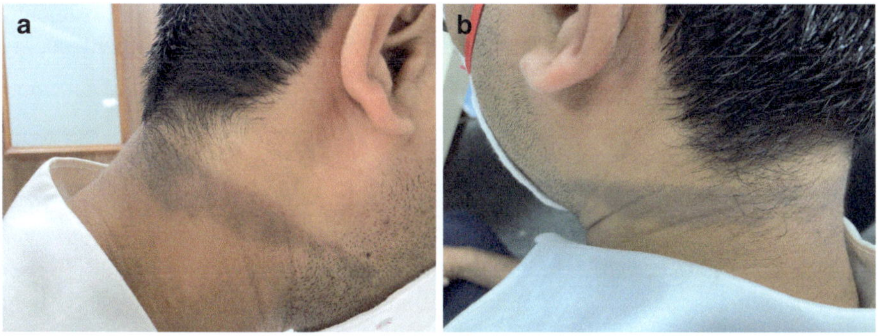

Fig. 12.12 (**a**, **b**) Noneczematous pigmented contact dermatitis. Linear band of hyperpigmentation corresponding to the site of repeated friction with elastic loop of mask

name refers to the irritant contact dermatitis which involves the webspaces, interphalangeal joint creases, proximal nail fold, nail cuticle, and consequently the nails leading to brittle nails.

Green nail syndrome or chloronychia may develop due to infection by *P. aeruginosa*, probably as a consequence of colonization secondary to humidity due to prolonged wearing of gloves. Lastly, aggravation of pre-existing conditions such as acne, rosacea, perioral dermatitis, seborrheic dermatitis, and hand dermatitis has been noted, especially in healthcare workers [40].

The only measure which seems to help is *moisturization*. One should apply moisturizers liberally prior to donning mask and face shield, and hospitals are advised to switch to alcohol-based handrub with moisturizing factors in it [41].

12.5 Skin Manifestations After COVID-19 Vaccination

Postvaccination cutaneous adverse events can be seen in about 10–30% of vaccine recipients according to a summary of clinical trial data of the approved vaccines, mostly local site reactions [42]. A similar number was seen in a real-life recipient-reported study of 867 Iranian residents, including those who had received Covaxin and AstraZeneca (Covishield) [43]. The common cutaneous adverse events seen with all COVID-19 vaccines include local site injection reaction (1–15%), maculopapular exanthem (3.5–5%), and urticaria (2.5–5%). They are transient, usually resolving within a week; rarely, urticarial lesions may continue to appear for 12–16 weeks.

Other reported cutaneous adverse events include urticarial vasculitis, perniosis, pityriasis rosea, erythema multiforme-like lesions, erythromelalgia, and petechiae. Triggering of some diseases such as lichen planus, lichen planopilaris (Pfizer, AstraZeneca), pityriasis rubra pilaris, guttate psoriasis (Pfizer), and alopecia areata (Pfizer/Moderna) has also been reported [44, 45]. These usually start within a week and may occur, for the first time, up to 16 weeks after the first, second, or third dose.

Post-vaccine reactivation of varicella-zoster virus leading to herpes zoster has been reported with all COVID-19 vaccines, although the exact incidence is not known.

12.6 Conclusion

COVID-19 infection can affect every system, and many of these are identified after the acute symptoms have subsided. The skin and mucosae represent a visible aspect of the consequences of systemic inflammation; and while this may potentially help diagnosticians, it also means more psychological distress for the patient, especially with hair loss and nail plate changes. Adverse skin changes due to use of personal protective equipment lead to minor but persistent problems for healthcare workers who are already under extreme work stress; they must be prevented, identified, and promptly addressed.

References

1. Visconti A, Bataille V, Rossi N, Kluk J, Murphy R, Puig S, et al. Diagnostic value of cutaneous manifestation of SARS-CoV-2 infection. Br J Dermatol. 2021;184:880–7.
2. Rerknimitr P, Theerawattanawit C, Lertpichitkul P, Jan-Tarabenjakul W, Putcharoen O, Puthanakit T, et al. Skin manifestations in COVID-19: the tropics experience. J Dermatol. 2020;47:444–6.
3. Matar S, Oulès B, Sohier P, Chosidow O, Beylot-Barroy M, Dupin N, et al. Cutaneous manifestations in SARS-CoV-2 infection (COVID-19): a French experience and a systematic review of the literature. J Eur Acad Dermatol Venereol. 2020;34:686–9.
4. Solak EO, Ketencioglu BB, Aslaner H, Cinar SL, Kartal D, Benli AR, et al. Cutaneous symptoms of patients diagnosed with COVID-19 in one province: a cross-sectional survey. J Eur Acad Dermatol Venereol. 2021;35:105–6.
5. Tammaro A, Adebanjo GAR, Parisella FR, Pezzuto A, Rello J. Cutaneous manifestations in COVID-19: the experiences of Barcelona and Rome. J Eur Acad Dermatol Venereol. 2020;34:306–7.
6. Tamai M, Maekawa A, Goto N, Ge L, Nishida T, Iwahashi H, et al. Three cases of COVID-19 patients presenting with erythema. J Dermatol. 2020;47:1175–8.
7. Pangti R, Gupta S, Nischal N, Trikha A. Recognizable vascular skin manifestations of SARS-CoV-2 (COVID-19) infection are uncommon in patients with darker skin phototypes. Clin Exp Dermatol. 2021;46:180–2.
8. Fernandez-Nieto D, Ortega-Quijano D, Suarez-Valle A, Jimenez-Cauhe J, Jaen-Olasolo P, Fernandez-Guarino M. Lack of skin manifestations in COVID-19 hospitalized patients during the second epidemic wave in Spain: a possible association with a novel SARS-CoV-2 variant—a cross-sectional study. J Eur Acad Dermatol Venereol. 2021;35:e183–5.
9. Sardana K, Sinha S, Yadav A, Deepak D, Panesar S, Mathachan SR. Paucity of cutaneous manifestations of COVID-19 among inpatients in a referral hospital in India. JAAD Int. 2022;8:10–5. https://doi.org/10.1016/j.jdin.2022.01.001.
10. Khurana A, Mittal A, Jain R, Mishra A, Mathachan SR. Rarity of cutaneous findings among asymptomatic to mildly symptomatic patients with COVID-19 admitted to a COVID care facility in Delhi, India: an observational study. Br J Dermatol. 2021;185:666–7.
11. Jamshidi P, Hajikhani B, Mirsaeidi M, Vahidnezhad H, Dadashi M, Nasiri MJ. Skin manifestations in COVID-19 patients: are they indicators for disease severity? A systematic review. Front Med (Lausanne). 2021;8:634208.

12. Gisondi P, Leo SD, Bellinato F, Cazzaniga S, Piaserico S, Naldi L. Time of onset of selected skin lesions associated with COVID-19: a systematic review. Dermatol Ther (Heidelb). 2021;11:695–705.
13. Unterluggauer L, Pospischil I, Krall C, et al. Cutaneous manifestations of SARS-CoV-2: a 2-center, prospective, case-controlled study. J Am Acad Dermatol. 2021;85(1):202–4.
14. Ng SM. Prolonged dermatological manifestation 4 weeks following recovery of COVID-19 in a child. BMJ Case Rep. 2020;13:e237056.
15. Bourgonje AR, Abdulle AE, Timens W, Hillebrands JL, Navis GJ, Gordijn SJ, et al. Angiotensin-converting enzyme 2 (ACE2), SARS-CoV-2 and the pathophysiology of coronavirus disease 2019 (COVID-19). J Pathol. 2020;251:228–48.
16. Suchonwanit P, Leerunyakul K, Kositkuljorn C. Cutaneous manifestations in COVID-19: lessons learned from current evidence. J Am Acad Dermatol. 2020;83:57–60.
17. Jamiolkowski D, Mühleisen B, Müller S, Navarini AA, Tzankov A, Roider E. SARS-CoV-2 PCR testing of skin for COVID-19 diagnostics: a case report. Lancet. 2020;396:598–9.
18. Colmenero I, Santonja C, Alonso-Riaño M, Noguera-Morel L, Hernández-Martín A, Andina D, et al. SARS-CoV-2 endothelial infection causes COVID-19 chilblains: histopathological, immunohistochemical and ultrastructural study of seven paediatric cases. Br J Dermatol. 2020;183:729–37.
19. Seque CA, Enokihara MMSES, Porro AM, Tomimori J. Skin manifestations associated with COVID-19. An Bras Dermatol. 2022;97(1):75–88.
20. Keshavarz P, Yazdanpanah F, Azhdari S, Kavandi H, Nikeghbal P, Bazyar A, Rafiee F, Nejati SF, Sadabad FE, Rezaei N. Coronavirus disease 2019 (COVID-19): a systematic review of 133 children that presented with Kawasaki-like multisystem inflammatory syndrome. J Med Virol. 2021;93:5458–73.
21. Esmaeilzadeh H, Mortazavi N, Salehi A, Fatemian H, Dehghani SM, Vali M, Vardanjani HM. Effect of COVID-19 on Kawasaki disease: decrease age of onset and increase skin manifestation. BMC Pediatr. 2021;21:571.
22. Freeman EE, McMahon DE, Lipoff JB, Rosenbach M, Kovarik C, Desai SR, Harp J, Takeshita J, French LE, Lim HW, Thiers BH, Hruza GJ, Fox LP. The spectrum of COVID-19-associated dermatologic manifestations: an international registry of 716 patients from 31 countries. J Am Acad Dermatol. 2020;83:1118–29.
23. Nuno-Gonzalez A, Martin-Carrillo P, Magaletsky K, Rios MDM, Mañas CH, Almazan JA, et al. Prevalence of mucocutaneous manifestations in 666 patients with COVID-19 in a field hospital in Spain: oral and palmoplantar findings. Br J Dermatol. 2021;184:184–5.
24. Starace M, Iorizzo M, Sechi A, Alessandrini AM, Carpanese M, Bruni F, et al. Trichodynia and telogen effluvium in COVID-19 patients: results of an international expert opinion survey on diagnosis and management. JAAD Int. 2021;5:11–8.
25. Hussain N, Agarwala P, Iqbal K, Omar HMS, Jangid G, Patel V, et al. A systematic review of acute telogen effluvium, a harrowing post-COVID-19 manifestation. J Med Virol. 2021; https://doi.org/10.1002/jmv.27534.
26. Abrantes TF, Artounian KA, Falsey R, Simão JCL, Vañó-Galván S, Ferreira SB, Davis TL, Ridenour W, Goren A, Tosti A, Wambier CG. Time of onset and duration of post-COVID-19 acute telogen effluvium. J Am Acad Dermatol. 2021;85:975–6.
27. Moreno-Arrones OM, Lobato-Berezo A, Gomez-Zubiaur A. SARS-CoV-2-induced telogen effluvium: a multicentric study. J Eur Acad Dermatol Venereol. 2021;35:e181–3.
28. Sattur SS, Sattur IS. COVID-19 infection: impact on hair. Indian J Plast Surg. 2021;54:521–6.
29. Aksoy H, Yıldırım UM, Ergen P, Gürel MS. COVID-19 induced telogen effluvium. Dermatol Ther. 2021;34:e15175.
30. Thuangtong R, Angkasekwinai N, Leeyaphan C, et al. Patient recovery from COVID-19 infections: follow-up of hair, nail, and cutaneous manifestations. Biomed Res Int. 2021;2021:5595016.
31. Preda-Naumescu A, Penney K, Pearlman RL, Brodell RT, Daniel CR, Nahar VK. Nail manifestations in COVID-19: insight into a systemic viral disease. Skin Appendage Disord. 2021;183:1–6.

32. Hadeler E, Morrison BW, Tosti A. A review of nail findings associated with COVID-19 infection. J Eur Acad Dermatol Venereol. 2021;35:e699–709.
33. Neri I, Guglielmo A, Virdi A, Gaspari V, Starace M, Piraccini BM. The red half-moon nail sign: a novel manifestation of coronavirus infection. J Eur Acad Dermatol Venereol. 2020;34:e663–5.
34. Martinez-Lopez A, Cuenca-Barrales C, Montero-Vilchez T, Molina-Leyva A, Arias-Santiago S. Review of adverse cutaneous reactions of pharmacologic interventions for COVID-19: a guide for the dermatologist. J Am Acad Dermatol. 2020;83:1738–48.
35. Mohseni Afshar Z, Babazadeh A, Hasanpour A, Barary M, Sayad B, Janbakhsh A, Aryanian Z, Ebrahimpour S. Dermatological manifestations associated with COVID-19: a comprehensive review of the current knowledge. J Med Virol. 2021;93:5756–67.
36. Jose S, Cyriac MC, Dhandapani M. Health problems and skin damages caused by personal protective equipment: experience of frontline nurses caring for critical COVID-19 patients in intensive care units. Indian J Crit Care Med. 2021;25:134–9.
37. Etgu F, Onder S. Skin problems related to personal protective equipment among healthcare workers during the COVID-19 pandemic (online research). Cutan Ocul Toxicol. 2021;40:207–13.
38. Teo WL. Diagnostic and management considerations for “maskne” in the era of COVID-19. J Am Acad Dermatol. 2021;84:520–1.
39. Kaul S, Kaur I, Jakhar D. Facial mask-related acne and acneiform eruption during the coronavirus disease 2019 pandemic: a case series. J Clin Aesthet Dermatol. 2021;14:32–4.
40. Chiriac AE, Chiriac A, Wollina U. Chloronychia in healthcare workers in COVID-19 times. Skin Appendage Disord. 2021;7:80–1.
41. Rivers JK, Arlette JP, DeKoven J, Guenther LC, Muhn C, Richer V, Rosen N, Tremblay JF, Wiseman MC, Zip C, Zloty D. Skin care and hygiene among healthcare professionals during and after the SARS-CoV-2 pandemic. SAGE Open Med. 2021;8(9):20503121211062795. https://doi.org/10.1177/20503121211062795.
42. Sun Q, Fathy R, McMahon DE, Freeman EE. COVID-19 vaccines and the skin: the landscape of cutaneous vaccine reactions worldwide. Dermatol Clin. 2021;39:653–73.
43. Zare H, Rezapour H, Mahmoodzadeh S, Fereidouni M. Prevalence of COVID-19 vaccines (Sputnik V, AZD-1222, and Covaxin) side effects among healthcare workers in Birjand city. Iran Int Immunopharmacol. 2021;101:108351.
44. Diab R, Araghi F, Gheisari M, Kani ZA, Moravvej H. Lichen planus and lichen planopilaris flare after COVID-19 vaccination. Dermatol Ther. 2021;24:e15283. https://doi.org/10.1111/dth.15283.
45. Scollan ME, Breneman A, Kinariwalla N, Soliman Y, Youssef S, Bordone LA, Gallitano SM. Alopecia areata after SARS-CoV-2 vaccination. JAAD Case Rep. 2022;20:1–5.

Eye Complications Following COVID-19

13

Rohit Saxena and Rebika Dhiman

13.1 Introduction

Coronavirus disease (COVID-19) caused by severe acute respiratory syndrome coronavirus 2 (SARS-CoV-2) is an ongoing global pandemic. Earlier believed to be primarily a respiratory disease, COVID-19 has now been recognized as a multisystem disorder. Eye complications are being increasingly reported in the acute as well as recovery phase of the disease. This chapter outlines various ocular manifestations that have been reported in association with COVID-19 during and following the infection. The knowledge and understanding of these ocular manifestations is important to raise awareness about keeping COVID-19 as a differential in such cases, especially during the pandemic. This is crucial for the comprehensive management of the disease and entails adopting preventive measures for the safety of the examining clinician, who may be the first point of contact. The latter is important as Dr. Li Wenliang, an ophthalmologist, one of the first doctors who warned about the outbreak of COVID-19, died after becoming infected with SARS-CoV-2 in Wuhan, China, on February 7, 2020, at the young age of 33 years. He contracted the virus from an asymptomatic glaucoma patient in early January due to the close association with the patient during the ocular examination.

13.2 Pathophysiology

There are several proposed mechanisms for eye manifestations in SARS-CoV-2 infection.

R. Saxena (✉) · R. Dhiman
Dr. Rajendra Prasad Centre for Ophthalmic Sciences, All India Institute of Medical Sciences, New Delhi, India

A. Mohan, S. Mittal (eds.), *Post COVID-19 Complications and Management*, https://doi.org/10.1007/978-981-19-4407-9_13

The first hypothesis is the direct viral invasion in the tissue via angiotensin-converting enzyme-2 (ACE-2) receptor that acts as the primary functional receptor for the virus. Viral entry is facilitated by the binding of viral spike (S) protein to ACE-2 receptors. Thereafter, viral uptake and membrane fusion is promoted by priming of S protein by the host cellular transmembrane protease serine 2 (TMPRSS2). ACE-2 expression has been noted in several tissues, including the lungs, nasopharynx, heart, brain, and blood vessels. Several ocular structures express ACE-2 receptors and evidence supports the presence of ACE-2 and TMPRSS2 on ocular surface as well. This explains the tropism of SARS-CoV-2 for the ocular surface, suggesting that the eye may act as a conduit for viral entry in humans.

The second hypothesis is related to endothelial dysfunction and coagulopathy. This theory is supported by the presence of ACE-2 receptors on the endothelial cells that can lead to endothelial abnormalities such as endothelitis and microvascular dysfunction causing vasoconstriction, ischemia, and tissue edema. The heightened immune response causes increased levels of pro-inflammatory cytokines, in turn leading to hypercoagulability. This predisposes affected individuals to thrombotic events.

Thirdly, the exaggerated or dysregulated immune response-induced autoantibody production has been associated with the fresh occurrence of autoimmune disorders like antibody-positive optic neuritis, Miller Fisher syndrome, or myasthenia gravis. Autoantibody production occurs due to molecular mimicry in which viral antigens induce an immune response against self-proteins [1].

Lastly, SARS-CoV-2 pneumonia and respiratory insufficiency can lead to hypoxia-induced brain injury that may cause various neuro-ophthalmic manifestations.

13.3 Ocular and Extraocular Manifestations of COVID-19

COVID-19 may involve any part of the eye- the ocular surface, intraocular, or extraocular or may have neuro-ophthalmic manifestations. Vaccine-related ocular complications are also described. All these features have been summarized in Table 13.1.

1. *The ocular surface and cornea*

   Conjunctivitis is the most common ophthalmic involvement reported with COVID-19 infection. As discussed earlier, the ocular surface may also be the source of entry or dissemination of the virus. Various studies have reported conjunctival involvement in the range of 0.8–32% [2]. Hand-eye contact has been noted as a risk factor predisposing to conjunctival symptoms in COVID-19. Although the virus yield from the conjunctival samples has been poor on reverse transcriptase-polymerase chain reaction (RT-PCR), ocular surface is still considered the likely entry portal for the SARS-CoV-2.

   Conjunctival hyperemia, chemosis, epiphora, ocular irritation, foreign body sensation, follicular conjunctivitis, and increased secretions are commonly

Table 13.1 Summary of eye manifestations in COVID-19

S. no.	Structure involved	Type of involvement
1	Ocular surface and cornea	(a) Conjunctivitis—follicular, hemorrhagic, pseudomembranous (b) Conjunctival hyperemia (c) Chemosis (d) Epiphora (e) Foreign body sensation (f) Episcleritis
2	Intraocular	(a) Uveitis—anterior, intermediate, and posterior (b) CRVO (c) CRAO (d) Other retinal abnormalities—acute retinal necrosis (ARN), acute macular neuroretinopathy (AMN), paracentral acute middle maculopathy (PAMM), etc.
3	Extraocular	(a) Eyelid abnormalities—blepharitis, lid margin hyperemia/ telangiectasia, meibomian orifice problems (b) Acute dacryoadenitis (c) Orbital cellulitis and sinusitis (d) Rhino-orbital-cerebral mucormycosis
4	Neuro-ophthalmic	(a) Optic neuritis (b) Idiopathic intracranial hypertension (IIH) (c) Cranial neuropathy (d) Posterior reversible encephalopathy syndrome (PRES) (e) Ischemic optic neuropathy—arteritic and non-arteritic AION (f) Cortical visual impairment (CVI) (g) Multisystem inflammatory syndrome in children (MIS-C) (h) Myasthenia gravis (i) Nystagmus and other eye movement disorders (j) Pupillary abnormalities
5	Vaccine-related	(a) Mild ocular features—episcleritis, anterior scleritis, acute macular neuroretinopathy, paracentral acute middle maculopathy, and subretinal fluid (b) Transient vision loss or visual field defects (c) CRVO (d) Optic neuritis (e) Exacerbation of VKH (f) Myasthenia gravis (g) Acute macular neuroretinopathy (h) Central serous retinopathy (i) Uveitis (j) Multiple evanescent white dot syndrome and cranial nerve palsies

described features. Most cases of follicular conjunctivitis have been reported in the subacute phase of the disease, i.e., the second week. Conjunctival involvement has occasionally been seen as the presenting symptom of the disease, with patients developing other respiratory signs of SARS-CoV-2 a few days later. Rarely, it may be the sole manifestation of the disease. Conjunctivitis has also been reported in the late or recovery phase of SARS-CoV-2 infection. Early-onset conjunctivitis is attributed to direct viral invasion and involves treatment with topical antibiotics. On the other hand, late-onset conjunctivitis is presumably an immune-mediated response. This has more severe manifestations such as bilateral involvement and corneal involvement and needs treatment with topical steroids and lubricants. Ribavirin has been used in some cases. Hemorrhagic and pseudomembranous forms of conjunctivitis have also been reported where a complete resolution was noted with topical antibiotics, steroids, and daily debridement of the pseudomembrane [3].

Conjunctivitis has also been seen as a manifestation of the multisystem inflammatory syndrome in children (MIS-C) that is reported to occur a few weeks after SARS-CoV-2 infection and bears a resemblance to Kawasaki disease. It is related to delayed immune response occurring following COVID-19 and is associated with elevated inflammatory markers.

Episcleritis is another rare manifestation of COVID-19 infection and is infrequently seen as a presenting symptom. It is usually self-limiting and requires no specific therapy.

2. *Intraocular*
   (a) Uveitis—All forms of uveitis, i.e., anterior, intermediate, and posterior, have been described during the course of the disease.
   (b) Posterior segment
      (i) Venous occlusions—Inflammatory reaction and hypercoagulability seen with COVID-19 infection may lead to venous occlusions (Fig. 13.1). There are several reports of unilateral or bilateral central retinal vein occlusion (CRVO) and impending CRVO following COVID-19 infection in young as well as elderly individuals. Usually good visual recovery has been noted with steroids and anticoagulants. Cases with macular involvement need anti-VEGF treatment. Papillophlebitis, a milder form of CRVO, has been noted either as a manifestation of COVID-19 or as a consequence of prone positioning in ICU patients admitted for management of COVID-19. Prone positioning causes direct compression on the eye, increases orbital venous pressure, and consequently increases intraocular pressure. Therefore, fundus examination becomes necessary in prone-positioned ICU patients. Also, protective cushioning of the eyes and maintaining the head position above heart level are some preventive measures that must be implemented [4].
      (ii) Arterial occlusion—Central retinal artery occlusion (CRAO) is less commonly reported than CRVO in COVID-19. It is a blinding condition that has been linked with elevated inflammatory markers like interleukin-6, C-Reactive Protein (CRP), ferritin, D-dimer, and fibrinogen. Rarely, combined CRVO and CRAO can also be seen.
      (iii) Other retinal abnormalities
         1. Acute retinal necrosis (ARN) is a rare manifestation of COVID-19.
         2. Acute macular neuroretinopathy (AMN) and paracentral acute middle maculopathy (PAMM).

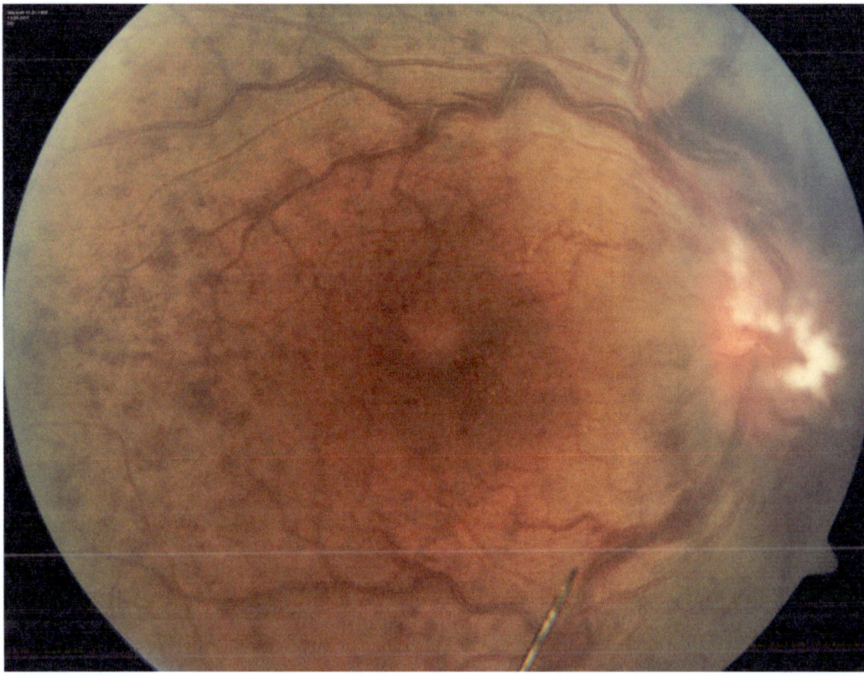

Fig. 13.1 Fundus photograph of a 55-year-old male showing right-sided central retinal venous occlusion noted a week after being diagnosed with COVID-19

3. Subclinical abnormalities on optical coherence tomography (OCT) in the retinal layers like bilateral hyperreflectivity in several layers of the retina that are more prominent at the papillomacular bundle, disruption of the ellipsoid zone and interdigitation zone, and loss of inner nuclear layer (INL) volume have been described.
4. Vitritis can be seen but should be diagnosed after ruling out other infectious causes.
5. Nonspecific retinal changes like peripapillary and peripheral retinal hemorrhages, cotton-wool spots, hard exudates, dilated veins, tortuous vessels, and macular pigmentation have been noted.
6. OCT angiography (OCT-A) has shown significant, diffuse perfusion loss in several areas of the post COVID 19 patients' retinas compared with healthy eyes.
7. On Fluid Attenuated Inversion Recovery (FLAIR) weighted images, abnormal magnetic resonance imaging (MRI) findings have been seen at the posterior pole in few patients with COVID-19 consisting of one or several hyperintense nodules in the macular region. These lesions are postulated to be either direct inflammatory infiltration of the retina or microangiopathic disease from viral infection.

(iv) Choroidal abnormalities—Reactivation of serpiginous choroiditis has been reported following COVID-19 infection. Other differentials like tuberculosis, hepatitis B and C, human immunodeficiency virus (HIV), and syphilis should be ruled out before initiating immunomodulatory therapy.

3. *Extraocular*
   (a) Lid—Eyelid abnormalities in the form of meibomian orifice problems and lid margin hyperemia/telangiectasia may be seen. Blepharitis is seen as a late manifestation of the disease.
   (b) Orbital—Orbital manifestations may vary from non-specific retro-orbital pain to life-threatening invasive mucormycosis.
      (i) Acute dacryoadenitis as a late complication of SARS-CoV-2 has been reported in a patient otherwise devoid of any COVID-19 symptoms and later detected positive for SARS-CoV-2 antibodies. Retrograde spread of the virus to the lacrimal gland via the ductules or immunologic response to the gland are the possible mechanisms.
      (ii) Orbital cellulitis and sinusitis—Orbital cellulitis has been seen in young patients presenting as progressive painful orbital swelling in the absence of any chronic sinus disease. Orbital abscess with globe perforation has also been reported.
      (iii) Rhino-orbital-cerebral mucormycosis (Fig. 13.2) is a life-threatening opportunistic infection that is increasingly reported with moderate to severe COVID-19 infection. The risk factors are the presence of associated comorbidities like uncontrolled diabetes, diabetic ketoacidosis and corticosteroid use for the management of COVID-19. Facial or orbital pain, headache, periocular swelling, double vision, and diminution of vision may be the early features of the disease. In suspected cases, clinical assessment of vision, pupillary reactions, and ocular motility should be done. Nasal swab for KOH mount and cultures should be sent to confirm the diagnosis. Neuroimaging is useful in assessing the extent of the disease. Aggressive management with intravenous liposomal amphotericin B with or without surgical debridement, along with strict glycemic control, is required. The reported

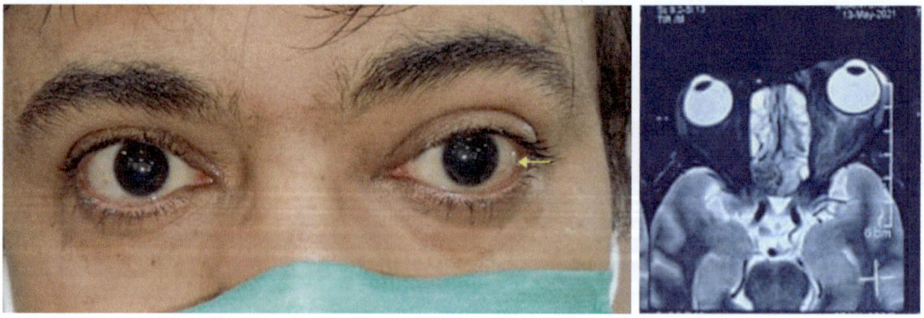

Fig. 13.2 Left-sided conjunctival congestion with mild proptosis noted in a patient post-COVID-19. MRI image showing diffuse orbital involvement of the left side suggestive of orbital mucormycosis

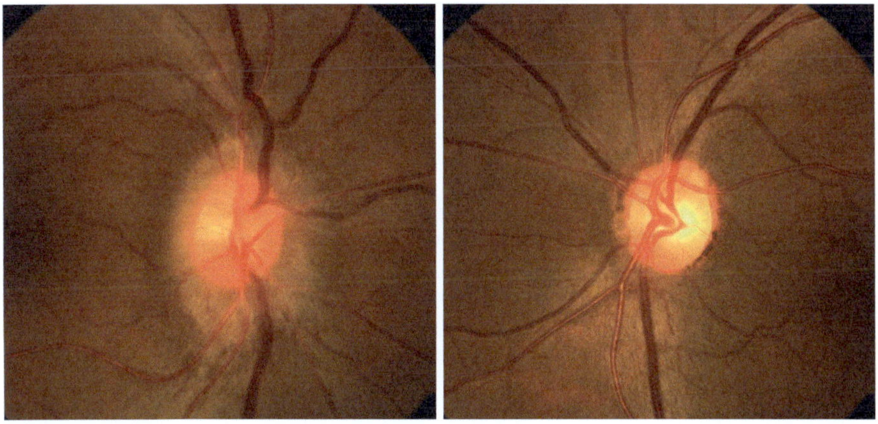

Fig. 13.3 Right-sided optic neuritis noted in a 50-year-old female patient 1 month after COVID-19 infection. Visual acuity on presentation was the perception of light in the right eye. The patient was tested positive for MOG antibody and responded well to steroids

mortality despite treatment is as high as 50%, and therefore, early diagnosis and management is imperative [3, 5].

4. *Neuro-ophthalmic manifestations*—Various neuro-ophthalmic manifestations have been documented in association with COVID-19 infection.
   (a) Optic neuritis (Fig. 13.3)

   There are several reports of unilateral or bilateral optic neuritis during the course or following recovery of COVID-19 infection. Para- and post-infectious demyelinating syndromes are known to occur following viral illnesses. So, the occurrence of optic neuritis in association with COVID-19 may be explained by a similar demyelinating process that is initiated either by the exposure to viral antigens related to viral neurotropism or by autoantibody production. The clinical presentation could be typical, with periventricular demyelinating lesions on MRI in a young female patient suggestive of multiple sclerosis (MS), or maybe atypical with myelitis and myelin oligodendrocyte (MOG) or anti-AQP4 (NMO) antibody positivity. Optic neuritis may occur as a presenting feature of COVID-19. Usually, good visual recovery has been noted with intravenous methylprednisolone (IVMP) and/or plasma exchange (PLEX). However, other infectious and inflammatory causes should be excluded.

   Panuveitis and optic neuritis as a presenting feature have also been reported. The simultaneous occurrence of uveitis and optic neuritis is explained by the presence of ACE-2 receptors in both the ocular tissues—choroid as well as central nervous system (CNS) [6].

   Acute disseminated encephalomyelitis (ADEM) presenting with bilateral vision loss and sensory deficit is also known [7]. The diagnosis was made based on neuroimaging showing multiple T1 post gadolinium-enhancing lesions in the brain, lesion in the spinal cord, and bilateral optic nerve

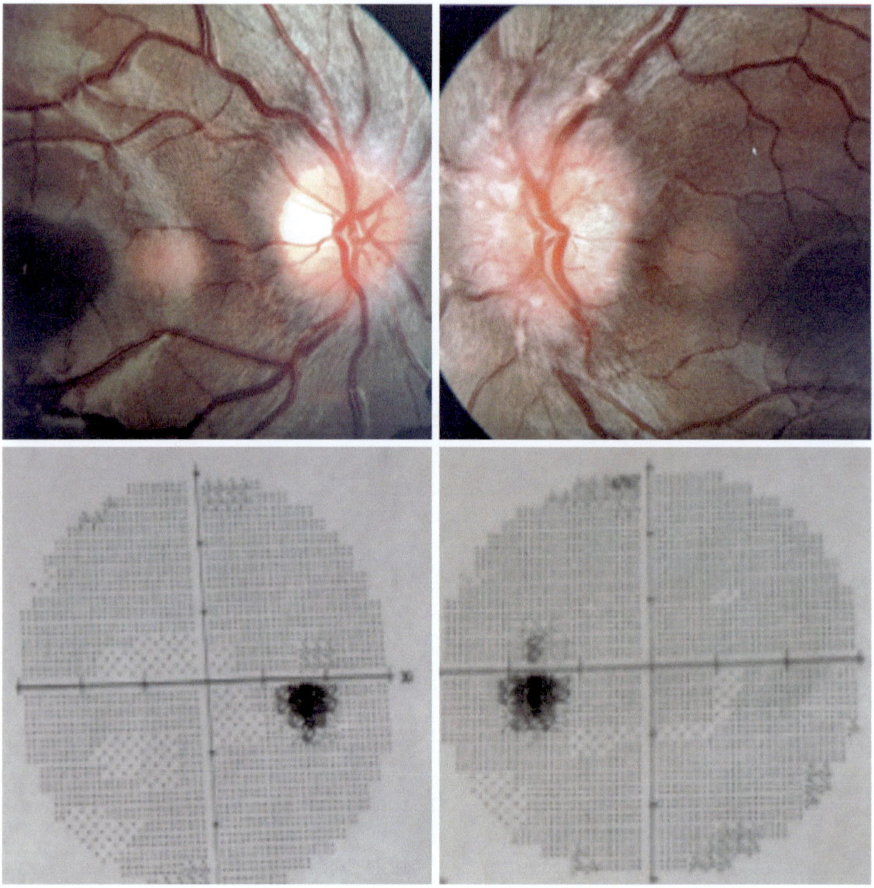

Fig. 13.4 Papilledema in a young female patient a month after being tested positive for SARS-CoV-2. Visual fields show mild enlargement of the blind spot, and neuroimaging was normal suggestive of idiopathic intracranial hypertension

enhancement. Significant visual recovery was noted after management with IVMP and IV immunoglobulins.

(b) Idiopathic intracranial hypertension (IIH)

There are reports of fresh-onset headache with raised intracranial pressure (defined as CSF opening pressure > 250 mm of H_2O) without encephalitis or meningitis following COVID-19 infection. However, disc edema may not be noted in all cases. Idiopathic intracranial hypertension with disc edema may be a presenting feature in COVID-19 and is also seen during the recovery phase (Fig. 13.4). Recovery of visual complaints and field defects occurs with lowering the CSF pressures with acetazolamide therapy. IIH is possibly caused by venous congestion due to low-grade inflammation and

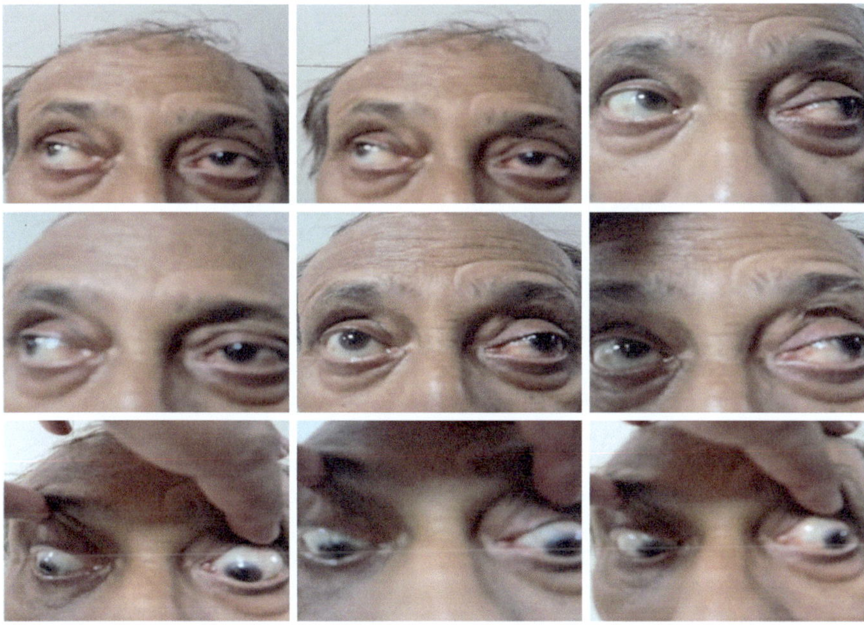

Fig. 13.5 Left-sided third nerve palsy showing drooping of the lids and limitation of adduction, elevation, and depression in an elderly patient with uncontrolled diabetic status. RT-PCR was negative, and patient did not have any systemic features of COVID-19 infection. But IgG COVID-19 antibody titers were markedly elevated. Neuroimaging was unremarkable

with hypercoagulable state precipitated by COVID-19 infection, leading to hyperviscosity and less CSF absorption.

(c) Cranial neuropathy

Ocular motor palsies have been seen following COVID-19 infection either as an isolated pathology or a manifestation of underlying systemic disease like Miller Fisher syndrome. There are reports of oculomotor (Fig. 13.5), trochlear, abducent, and facial palsy with COVID-19. While some patients had pre-existing vascular comorbidities, others were healthy young adults.

Acute demyelinating inflammatory polyneuropathy leading to third nerve and abducent nerve palsy has also been reported, likely due to the virus-mediated immune response. MRI findings may include enhancement of the optic nerve sheath and posterior Tenon's capsule, which may be due to viral leptomeningeal invasion or an ischemic process [8].

Guillain-Barre syndrome (GBS) presenting with facial paresis or diplegia, Miller Fisher syndrome with features of anosmia, ageusia, internuclear ophthalmoparesis, fascicular oculomotor palsy, ataxia, areflexia, albuminocytologic dissociation, GD1b-IgG antibody positivity and polyneuritis cranialis with ageusia, bilateral abducens palsy, areflexia, and albumino-cytologic dissociation are some other manifestations of COVID-19 infection. Good recovery has been demonstrated with treatment in most cases [9].

(d) Posterior reversible encephalopathy syndrome (PRES)

PRES is a neurological disorder characterized by vasogenic edema with a distinctive parieto-occipital involvement evident on neuroimaging. PRES has been reported in elderly patients with severe COVID-19 infection requiring intensive care unit (ICU) care with respiratory support. The patients usually present with seizures and occasionally with neuro-ophthalmic manifestations like visual field defects, cortical blindness, and visual hallucinations. There is also a report of hallucinatory palinopsia, the persistent recurrence of a visual image after the stimulus has been removed [10]. Cytokine storm, endothelial abnormalities, and SARS-CoV-2 pneumonia-related hypoxemia are the possible factors that affect cerebral autoregulation leading to cerebral vasodilatation, neuronal swelling, and vasogenic edema. Usually, good recovery has been noted in most cases.

(e) Ischemic optic neuropathy

Non-arteritic ischemic optic neuropathy (NAION) has been noted in already predisposed individuals, i.e., individuals with vascular comorbidities like diabetes and hypertension. Bilateral NAION has also been reported due to prone positioning in a patient with COVID-19-related acute respiratory distress syndrome (ARDS) [11]. Prone positioning is known to affect ocular perfusion and cause raised intraocular pressure. There are also rare reports of increasing presentation of giant cell arteritis (almost five-fold high) during the pandemic [12]. However, the cause-effect relationship could not be established definitively.

(f) Cortical visual impairment (CVI)

Greater incidence of stroke and younger age of incidence of stroke have been noted with SARS-CoV-2 infection than with other coronaviruses, influenza, or seasonal viruses. Coagulation disorders, endothelial abnormalities, and excessive inflammatory response are the causative factors. Therefore, early anticoagulation therapy is recommended in moderate-severe COVID-19.

Occipital and visual pathway involvement in stroke can lead to neuro-ophthalmic manifestations like vision loss and visual field defects.

(g) Multisystem inflammatory syndrome in children (MIS-C)

MIS-C is characterized by inflammation of multisystem organs like the heart, lungs, kidneys, brain, skin, eyes, or gastrointestinal organs ($\geq$2) and elevated inflammatory markers associated with recent SARS-CoV-2 infection. This is associated with an exaggerated immune response in children. Inflammatory markers like C-reactive protein (CRP), erythrocyte sedimentation rate (ESR), fibrinogen, procalcitonin, D-dimer, ferritin, lactic acid dehydrogenase (LDH), or interleukin-6 (IL-6) are elevated. Raised CSF pressures, related to altered CSF dynamics due to inflammatory or infectious meningitis, have been documented in the setting of MIS-C following

COVID-19 infection. Disc edema and abducent nerve palsy due to elevated intracranial pressure have been reported in some of these patients. Usually, the recovery is good with management.

(h) Myasthenia gravis

Exacerbation, as well as new cases of myasthenia gravis, may occur following COVID-19. The common presenting symptoms are diplopia and ptosis. The patients are positive for acetylcholinesterase (AchR) or muscle-specific tyrosine kinase (MuSK) antibodies and respond well to pyridostigmine.

(i) Nystagmus and other eye movement disorders

There are isolated reports of nystagmus and other eye movement disorders like intermittent horizontal nystagmus with a rotatory component [13], opsoclonus (rapid, chaotic, involuntary saccadic, multidirectional eye movements), and bilateral horizontal pendular nystagmus in COVID-19 patients [14].

(j) Pupillary abnormalities

Adie's pupil due to parasympathetic denervation following viral infections is not uncommon. Adie's tonic pupil has been documented in association with SARS-CoV-2 infection. Adie-Holmes syndrome with anisocoria and absence of deep tendon reflexes in upper and lower limbs has also been reported [15].

5. Vaccine-related complications

As the vaccination drive is ongoing, several COVID-19 vaccines have been introduced, such as RNA vaccines, DNA vaccines, and replication-defective viral vector vaccines. Subsequently, there have been reports of vaccine-related ocular complications. The mechanism of ocular disease post-vaccination can be an immunologic response to the spike antigen, other viral antigens, or components of adenovirus causing molecular mimicry.

Mild reversible ocular adverse events like episcleritis, anterior scleritis, acute macular neuroretinopathy, paracentral acute middle maculopathy, and subretinal fluid have been reported with inactivated COVID-19 vaccine. Thromboembolic events, including CRVO, have been noted with adenovirus vector-based COVID-19 vaccines. This has been attributed to systemic inflammation, platelet, and endothelial dysfunction. There have been rare cases of a transient decrease in vision and transient visual field defects. Occurrence of autoimmune diseases like bilateral arteritic anterior ischemic optic neuropathy (AAION) and bilateral acute zonal occult outer retinopathy (AZOOR) has been seen following vaccination suggesting cross-reactivity of neutralizing antibodies against SARS-CoV-2 spike proteins and host cell antigens [16].

There are numerous reports of postvaccination optic neuritis worldwide, some of whom were positive for myelin oligodendrocyte glycoprotein (MOG) antibodies [17]. Other noteworthy ocular events are Vogt-Koyanagi-Harada (VKH) disease exacerbation, myasthenia gravis, acute macular neuroretinopathy, central serous retinopathy, thrombosis, uveitis, multiple evanescent white dot syndrome, and cranial nerve palsies.

While multiple reports of side-effects following a vaccine injection have been documented, the mere temporal relationship does not necessarily prove causality. The reported frequency of the side effects is considered rare given the millions of people who have received one or more vaccines. The possible reasons for these effects may be related to potentially susceptible individuals exhibiting a maladaptive immune response. Vaccines have added adjuvants within them to boost the immunogenic efficacy, and these adjuvants potentiate the innate and adaptive immune response, which may lead to autoimmune or inflammatory conditions in a small group of persons.

13.4 Preventive Measures in Ophthalmic Practice

An ophthalmologist may be the first point of contact in SARS-CoV-2 infection due to these unusual ocular presentations. This necessitates the adherence to appropriate infection control measures based on the latest national and state health directives. Stratification of ophthalmic patients for clinical visits and utilization of tele-ophthalmology practices as much as possible for routine cases may be done. For outpatient examination, use of breath shields while using slit lamps, disinfection, and cleaning of instruments like tonometers, trial frames, pinhole occluders, and B-scan probes are advocated especially during the pandemic. Special care to cover the eyes, nose, and mouth with masks and face shields, use of gloves, and observing proper hand etiquette before and after patient examination are the key to prevent cross-transmission.

13.5 Conclusion

This chapter elaborates various eye manifestations of COVID-19. Considering the proximity required in the ophthalmic examination, understanding the ophthalmic manifestations of COVID-19 becomes important. Strict adherence to appropriate infection control measures while examining these patients will ensure the safety of the healthcare worker and the patients.

References

1. Tisdale AK, Dinkin M, Chwalisz BK. Afferent and efferent neuro-ophthalmic complications of coronavirus disease 19. J Neuroophthalmol. 2021;41:154–65.
2. Dhiman R, Rakheja V, Saxena R. An ophthalmologist's insight into the viral pandemics. J Optom. 2021;15(1):35–43. https://doi.org/10.1016/j.optom.2020.10.005.
3. Sen M, Honavar S, Sharma N, Sachdev M. COVID-19 and eye. Indian J Ophthalmol. 2021;69:488–509. https://doi.org/10.4103/ijo.IJO_297_21.
4. Sun L, Hymowitz M, Pomeranz HD. Eye protection for patients with COVID-19 undergoing prolonged prone-position ventilation. JAMA Ophthalmol. 2021;139:109–12. https://doi.org/10.1001/jamaophthalmol.2020.4988.

5. Singh AK, Singh R, Joshi SR, Misra A. Mucormycosis in COVID-19: a systematic review of cases reported worldwide and in India. Diabetes Metab Syndr. 2021;15(4):102146. https://doi.org/10.1016/j.dsx.2021.05.019.
6. Benito-Pascual B, Gegúndez JA, Díaz-Valle D, Arriola-Villalobos P, Carreño E, Culebras E, Rodríguez-Avial I, Benitez-Del-Castillo JM. Panuveitis and optic neuritis as a possible initial presentation of the novel coronavirus disease 2019 (COVID-19). Ocul Immunol Inflamm. 2020;28(6):922–5. https://doi.org/10.1080/09273948.2020.1792512.
7. Novi G, Rossi T, Pedemonte E, Saitta L, Rolla C, Roccatagliata L, Inglese M, Farinini D. Acute disseminated encephalomyelitis after SARS-CoV-2 infection. Neurol Neuroimmunol Neuroinflamm. 2020;7(5):e797. https://doi.org/10.1212/NXI.0000000000000797.
8. Dinkin M, Gao V, Kahan J, Bobker S, Simonetto M, Wechsler P, Harpe J, Greer C, Mints G, Salama G, Tsiouris AJ, Leifer D. COVID-19 presenting with ophthalmoparesis from cranial nerve palsy. Neurology. 2020;95(5):221–3. https://doi.org/10.1212/WNL.0000000000009700.
9. Gutierrez-Ortiz C, Mendez A, Rodrigo-Rey S, et al. Miller Fisher syndrome and polyneuritis cranialis in COVID-19. Neurology. 2020;95(5):e601–1212.
10. Ghosh R, Lahiri D, Dubey S, Ray BK, Benito-León J. Hallucinatory palinopsia in COVID-19-induced posterior reversible encephalopathy syndrome. J Neuroophthalmol. 2020;40(4):523–6. https://doi.org/10.1097/WNO.0000000000001135.
11. Clarke KM, Riga V, Shirodkar AL, et al. Proning related bilateral anterior ischaemic optic neuropathy in a patient with COVID-19 related acute respiratory distress syndrome. BMC Ophthalmol. 2021;21:276. https://doi.org/10.1186/s12886-021-02028-9.
12. Luther R, Skeoch S, Pauling JD, Curd C, Woodgate F, Tansley S. Increased number of cases of giant cell arteritis and higher rates of ophthalmic involvement during the era of COVID-19. Rheumatol Adv Pract. 2020;4(2):rkaa067. https://doi.org/10.1093/rap/rkaa067.
13. Ishaq II, Durrani T, Umar Z, Khan N, McCombe P, Ul Haq MA. Post-COVID opsoclonus myoclonus syndrome: a case report from Pakistan. Front Neurol. 2021;12:672524.
14. Pereira Coutinho M, Faustino P, Lourenço J, Leitão L. Acquired pendular nystagmus in the setting of COVID-19. Eur J Neurol. 2021;28(Suppl 1):767.
15. Kaya Tutar N, Kale N, Tugcu B. Adie-Holmes syndrome associated with COVID-19 ınfection. Indian J Ophthalmol. 2021;69(3):773–4.
16. Maleki A, Look-Why S, Manhapra A, Foster CS. COVID-19 recombinant mRNA vaccines and serious ocular inflammatory side effects: real or coincidence? J Ophthalmic Vis Res. 2021;16(3):490–501.
17. Alvarez LM, Neo YN, Davagnanam I, Ashenhurst M, Acheson J, Abdel-Hay A, et al. Post vaccination optic neuritis: observations from the SARS-CoV-2 pandemic. SSRN Electron J. https://doi.org/10.2139/ssrn.3889990.

Palliative Care Issues in Post-COVID-19

14

Raghav Gupta and Sushma Bhatnagar

Palliative care has been defined by the International Association for Hospice & Palliative Care (IAHPC) in 2018 as "The active, holistic care of individuals across all ages with serious health-related suffering due to severe illness, and especially of those near the end of life. It aims to improve the quality of life of patients and their caregivers" [1]. It is a multidimensional specialty that emphasizes the patient and family-based care and helps in symptomatic improvement of patients during the course of disease and treatment, as well as during the terminal stage when the focus is primarily comfort.

There is a common perception that palliative care is only for cancer patients, but in reality, it has spread its horizon and is required for critically ill [2] as well as patients suffering from chronic ailments. Globally, there is a constant gap between the clinical care required and the public healthcare infrastructure available. This gap came to the fore during the COVID pandemic. The pandemic has affected humankind at various levels—physical, psychological, socioeconomic, as well as spiritual. However, interdisciplinary coordination has given clinicians an opportunity to bridge the gap between clinical care and public healthcare measures. Recently, studies have emphasized the important role of palliative care in the pandemic [3, 4]. In fact, the need for palliative care has been felt not just during acute COVID but also during the post-COVID phase due to the myriad of symptoms that persist after recovery from acute illness.

It is now evident that a holistic approach is required to manage the post-COVID symptoms to provide a better quality of life for patients as well as caregivers. The role of the palliative care physician includes:

1. Symptomatic management, discussion about the course of illness, advanced care planning, and psychosocial support to the patient and family members [5, 6]

R. Gupta · S. Bhatnagar (✉)
Department of Onco-anesthesia and Palliative Medicine, AIIMS, New Delhi, India

A. Mohan, S. Mittal (eds.), *Post COVID-19 Complications and Management*,
https://doi.org/10.1007/978-981-19-4407-9_14

2. Teaching and training at the institute level to enable other colleagues to handle the increased demand for palliative care during the time of crisis [7]

14.1 Primary and Specialty Palliative Care

Any physician can provide primary palliative care. They can manage basic symptoms like pain, nausea, constipation, and anxiety. The role of a palliative care specialist was felt in the 1990s in order to provide specialist palliative care services for managing refractory symptoms, complex decision-making, and end-of-life care discussions. This assumes greater importance during a pandemic where many people are suffering at the same point of time [8].

14.2 Postulated Reasons for Post-COVID Symptoms

Several mechanisms have been proposed for the persistence of symptoms beyond the acute COVID episode, such as:

- The persistence of the virus in the body due to weak host immune response
- Relapse or reinfection
- An inflammatory reaction to the virus
- Deconditioning
- Anxiety and post-traumatic stress disorder

14.3 Post-COVID Symptoms

Majority of patients with COVID recover completely within a few days to a few weeks, but symptoms persist in a significant proportion.

These patients are often labeled as "long haulers" and the condition has been termed as post-COVID syndrome or "long COVID-19" [9]. Elderly and those affected by comorbidities are affected the most. Common signs and symptoms that are observed in post-COVID phase include:

- Fatigue and malaise
- Dyspnea
- Cough
- Chest pain
- Cognitive dysfunction including memory and concentration problems
- Insomnia
- Headache
- Palpitations
- Loss of smell or taste
- Depression and anxiety

- Fever
- Dizziness

14.4 Post-COVID Lung Sequelae

Post-COVID lung sequelae lead to breathlessness. This may be due to multiple causes. The Breathing-Thinking-Functioning model explains that inefficient breathing, thoughts about dying, and reduced body activity all together lead to breathlessness [10].

14.4.1 Non-pharmacological Management

- Blowing of a fan in front of the face
- Pursed lip breathing and prolonged exhalation
- Physiotherapy and rehabilitation
- Huff-puff technique to clear secretions
- Postural drainage

14.4.2 Pharmacological Management

- Anti-inflammatory and antiviral agents as per recommended guidelines.
- Anti-fibrotic agents, e.g., pirfenidone and nintedanib. No conclusive evidence is currently available for the beneficial role of these agents in post-COVID lung sequelae. The prescription of these drugs is to be decided on a case-to-case basis keeping risks as well as benefits in mind.
- Morphine given in low dose helps the patient with dyspnea and makes them cooperative while doing pulmonary physiotherapy.

14.5 Post-COVID Dyspnea: Management Principles

Dyspnea is one of the commonest post-COVID symptoms. The WHO recommends opioid use in refractory dyspnea.

- Oral and parenteral opioids have been shown to reduce the sensation of dyspnea without causing significant respiratory depression [11, 12]. Oral morphine can be given in the dose of 2.5 mg prn/q4h.
- Oral mirtazapine [13] in the dose of 15 mg once daily can be prescribed for post-COVID chronic dyspnea Alternatively, oral promethazine can be added in dosage of 25–50 mg thrice daily.

- A specialist palliative care physician should be involved in medical care if the above measures fail, for opioid-tolerant patients, and for patients with kidney or liver dysfunction.
- Non-pharmacological measures: cool wipes, menthol lozenges, cool room temperature, avoid fan due to potential aerosol generation, prone positioning, forward lean position, near window bed, and 20-min mindful breathing.

14.6 Post-COVID Cough: Management

- Codeine linctus (15–30 mg prn/QID) is the preferred first-line agent in the pharmacological management of COVID-associated chronic cough; oral morphine (2.5 mg prn/q4h) is used as the second-line agent [14]. Inhaled steroids and bronchodilators have also been tried in refractory cough with some benefit.
- Tiotropium (18 mcg daily) has also been used.
- Gabapentin (300 mg TDS up to a maximum dose of 600 mg TDS) or pregabalin (up to 150 mg BD) can be considered for refractory post-COVID cough [15].
- N-acetylcysteine (200 mg TDS up to the maximum dose of 600 mg BD) is useful in patients with productive cough with thick secretions.
- Non-pharmacological measures: Treat underlying causes, identify and avoid cough triggers (cold air, cold drinks, dry atmospheres, particular food and spices, exertion, talking), drink warm water and honey, and practice mindful coughing (surf the urge and huff if necessary); for productive cough, measures include huffing, incentive spirometry, and self-administered chest physiotherapy.

14.7 Post-COVID Fever

- Fever associated with headache or body ache is treated with oral paracetamol (1 g prn/QID) or ibuprofen (200–400 mg prn/QID).
- Non-pharmacological measures include rehydration, cool wipes, reducing room temperature, consuming cold drinks or ice cream, loose clothing, and light bedding.

14.8 Psychological and Spiritual Suffering

- Deep breathing exercises and relaxation techniques can be utilized.
- Benzodiazepines, e.g., alprazolam or lorazepam, should be used carefully in patients where anxiety is refractory to psychological measures. If required in elderly, these should be given in low dose and tapered rapidly [16].
- Second-line agents for the treatment of anxiety includes gabapentin, olanzapine, and haloperidol.
- Oral melatonin is an option for post-COVID patients with sleep disturbances [17].

14.9 Psychosocial Support

Post-COVID patients and caregivers both face challenges at the level of various fronts—physical, psychological, spiritual, and socioeconomic. Palliative care helps in alleviating the suffering at the physical and psychological levels. In general, communication with patients and caregivers regarding the disease course and prognosis is challenging, especially in terminal illnesses. This is even more difficult during the pandemic due to the need to maintain physical distancing and use of personal protective equipment. Palliative care plays an important role in solving this conundrum.

Healthcare providers need to:

- Give realistic hope and honest opinion
- Show empathy with the patient and their family members during the end stage of life
- Acknowledge the emotions demonstrated by the patient and family
- Listen patiently
- Handle any anger or dissatisfaction with maturity and restraint

Reports suggest that the mental health effects of COVID can persist for prolonged periods of time even after clinical recovery. Managing this stressful period is an essential aspect of palliative care [18].

14.10 Grief and Bereavement

Rapid deterioration in the health and a fatal outcome of COVID infection are events for which family members may not be mentally prepared. Due to policies of isolation, often the family members are unable to meet their loved ones in the last moments of life. In all these situations, palliative care plays an important role.

Management of grief and bereavement [19]:

1. Recognize the suffering and emotions of caregivers
2. Rule out organic causes such as psychiatric disorders
3. Provide psychological and emotional support
4. If required, refer to a mental healthcare professional

14.11 Psycho-education

The physician must give accurate information in a calm and composed manner during times of stress. Techniques such as yoga, meditation, mindful breathing, and problem-solving skills are extremely helpful. During end-of-life stage, if the patient requests, then spiritual concerns should be considered important and addressed, if possible. Therapies to foster purpose at the end of life will enhance the overall outcome. Pharmacological management in the form of escitalopram 10–20 mg/day or sertraline 50–200 mg/day can be prescribed for anxiety and depression. To overcome the anxiety due to the disease and disease-associated stigma, patients may be given lorazepam 1–2 mg at night. However, these drugs should be stopped at the earliest possible. Agitation or delirium may respond to haloperidol 2.5–5 mg/day or olanzapine 5–10 mg/day.

14.12 Take-Home Message

- Integration of palliative care in acute COVID and post-COVID phase is of paramount importance for enhanced decision-making, better symptom management, safe use of opioids, alleviation of social isolation at the end of life, and bereavement support. The knowledge and expertise of a palliative care specialist should be utilized for these purposes.
- One must optimize interdisciplinary coordination, maintain continuity of care, enhance social support, include palliative care services at the primary healthcare level with the help of teaching and training, and form standard treatment guidelines and protocol for different pandemic phases.

References

1. IAHPC. Global Consensus based palliative care definition. 2018. Houston, TX: The International Association for Hospice and Palliative Care. Retrieved from https://hospicecare.com/what-we-do/projects/consensus-based-definition-of-palliative-care/definition/
2. Aslakson R, Cheng J, Vollenweider D, et al. Evidence-based palliative care in the intensive care unit: a systematic review of interventions. J Palliat Med. 2014;17:219–35.
3. Radbruch L, Knaul FM, de Lima L, et al. The key role of palliative care in response to the COVID-19 tsunami of suffering. Lancet. 2020;395:1467–9.
4. Davies A, Hayes J. Palliative care in the context of a pandemic: similar but different. Clin Med (Lond). 2020;20:274–7.
5. Krakauer EL, Daubman B-R, Aloudat T, et al. Chap 2. Palliative care needs of people affected by natural hazards, political or ethnic conflict, epidemics of life-threatening infections, and other humanitarian crises. In: Waldman E, Glass M, editors. A field manual for palliative care in humanitarian crises. Oxford: Oxford University Press; 2019.
6. Arya A, Buchman S, Gagnon B, Downar J. Pandemic palliative care: beyond ventilators and saving lives. CMAJ. 2020;192(15):E400–4.
7. Downar J, Seccareccia D. Palliating a pandemic: "all patients must be cared for". J Pain Symptom Manag. 2010;39(2):291–5.
8. Quill TE, Abernethy AP. Generalist plus specialist palliative care—creating a more sustainable model. N Engl J Med. 2013;368(13):1173–5.
9. Carfì A, Bernabei R, Landi F. For the Gemelli against COVID-19 post-acute care study group. Persistent symptoms in patients after acute COVID-19. JAMA. 2020;324(6):603–5.
10. Spathis A, Burkin J, Moffat C, et al. Cutting through complexity: the breathing, thinking, functioning clinical model is an educational tool that facilitates chronic breathlessness management. NPJ Prim Care Respir Med. 2021;31:25.

11. Arroliga AC, Thompson BT, Ancukiewicz M, et al. Use of sedatives, opioids, and neuromuscular blocking agents in patients with acute lung injury and acute respiratory distress syndrome*. Crit Care Med. 2008;36(4):1083–8.
12. Serpa Neto A, Simonis FD, Barbas CSV, et al. Association between tidal volume size, duration of ventilation, and sedation needs in patients without acute respiratory distress syndrome: an individual patient data meta-analysis. Intensive Care Med. 2014;40(7):950–7.
13. Simon ST, Higginson IJ, Booth S, Harding R, Weingärtner V, Bausewein C. Benzodiazepines for the relief of breathlessness in advanced malignant and non-malignant diseases in adults. Cochrane Database Syst Rev. 2016;10:CD007354.
14. Treggiari MM, Romand J-A, Yanez DN, et al. Randomized trial of light versus deep sedation on mental health after critical illness*. Crit Care Med. 2009;37(9):2527.
15. Liu L, Wu AP, Yang Y, et al. Effects of Propofol on respiratory drive and patient-ventilator synchrony during pressure support ventilation in postoperative patients: a prospective study. Chin Med J. 2017;130(10):1155–60.
16. Subramanyam AA, Kedare J, Singh OP, Pinto C. Clinical practice guidelines for geriatric anxiety disorders. Indian J Psychiatry. 2018;60(suppl 3):S371–82.
17. Zhang R, Wang X, Ni L, et al. COVID-19: melatonin as a potential adjuvant treatment. Life Sci. 2020;250:117583. https://doi.org/10.1016/j.lfs.2020.117583.
18. Singhai P, Rao KS, Rao SR, Salins N. Palliative care for advanced cancer patients in the COVID-19 pandemic: challenges and adaptations. Cancer Res Stat Treat. 2020;3(Suppl S1):127–3.
19. Pallium India: e-book on palliative care guidelines for COVID-19. Available from https://www.palliumindia.org/cms/wp-content/uploads/2020/04/e-book-Palliative-Care-Guidelines-for COVID19 ver1.pdf. Last accessed on 2022 Feb 5.

MIX
Papier aus verantwortungsvollen Quellen
Paper from responsible sources
FSC® C105338

If you have any concerns about our products,
you can contact us on
ProductSafety@springernature.com

In case Publisher is established outside the EU,
the EU authorized representative is:
Springer Nature Customer Service Center GmbH
Europaplatz 3, 69115 Heidelberg, Germany

Printed by Libri Plureos GmbH
in Hamburg, Germany